Digestive Diseases –
Research and Clinical Developments Series

ULCERS: CAUSES, DIAGNOSIS, AND TREATMENT

DIGESTIVE DISEASES – RESEARCH AND CLINICAL DEVELOPMENTS SERIES

Effects, Diagnosis and Management of Extra-Esophageal Reflux
Nikki Johnston, Robert J. Toohill (Editors)
2010. ISBN 978-1-61668-177-7

Ulcers: Causes, Diagnosis, and Treatment
Danijel Erceg and Pero Milojeviæ (Editors)
2010. ISBN: 978-1-60741-253-3

Digestive Diseases –
Research and Clinical Developments Series

ULCERS: CAUSES, DIAGNOSIS, AND TREATMENT

DANIJEL ERCEG
AND
PERO MILOJEVIÆ
EDITORS

Nova Science Publishers, Inc.
New York

For permission to use material from this book please contact us:
Telephone 631-231-7269; Fax 631-231-8175
Web Site: http://www.novapublishers.com

LIBRARY OF CONGRESS CATALOGING-IN-PUBLICATION DATA

Ulcers : causes, diagnosis, and treatment / editors, Danijel Erceg and Pero Milojeviœ. p. ; cm.
Includes bibliographical references and index. ISBN 978-1-60741-253-3 (hardcover)
1. Peptic ulcer. 2. Digestive organs--Diseases. I. Erceg, Danijel. II. Milojeviœ, Pero., [DNLM: 1. Peptic Ulcer. 2. Ulcer. WI 350 U369 2009]
RC821.U443 2009, 616.3'43--dc22 2009037466

Published by Nova Science Publishers, Inc. ✢ New York

CONTENTS

PREFACE

An ulcer is the result of an imbalance between aggressive and defensive factors. The pathology of ulcer is complex and may involve overproduction of acid or pepsin, inadequate mucosal defense, reflux of bile and pancreatic juice into stomach. Peptic ulcer is a classical example of the biopsychosocial model of disease and like most diseases, it has a multifactorial origin. Furthermore, peptic ulcer disease (PUD) is one of the common disorders affecting the digestive system. The lifetime risk of ulcer is 5-10% in developed countries. This book examines the psychosocial risk factors for developing peptic ulcers. It is shown that PUD occurs more frequently among individuals with anxiety and depressive disorders.

The use of a fibrinogen- and thrombin-coated collagen patch for a perforated peptic ulcer is researched as a method to reduce morbidity and mortality rates. Through the application of such a device, previously used in hepatic surgery, a new and simple modification to the standard technique may improve the seal of the traditional repair, has no complications and makes the overall operation faster. In addition to peptic ulcers, the etiology, diagnosis and treatment of gastric and skin ulcers are explored in this book, including the four most common etiologies that account for the large majority of skin ulcers in the elderly, the prevention and treatment of pressure ulcers and the results of research done on opical opioid therapy in treating pain from ulcers.

Chapter 2 - Use of multiple non-steroidal anti-inflammatory drugs (NSAIDs) represents one of the risk factors for NSAID-associated peptic ulcer. However, insufficient evidence has been accumulated to conclude whether the risk of peptic ulcer increases with concomitant use of low-dose aspirin (L-aspirin) in long-term treatment with NSAID.

The majority of patients with rheumatoid arthritis (RA) display some of the risk factors for peptic ulcer and its complications. In addition, since long-term NSAID users, particularly RA patients, have a high risk of cardiovascular disease (CVD), determining the risk of peptic ulcer induced by NSAID alone or in combination with L-aspirin in the daily clinical setting of RA patients is essential. The primary objective of this study was to elucidate the risk of peptic ulcer induced by concomitant L-aspirin in Japanese RA outpatients on long-term NSAID treatment. Although endoscopic ulcer has been defined as an excavated mucosal break ≥3 mm in diameter in most studies, the clinical implications of endoscopic ulcers are unclear. A secondary objective was thus to evaluate whether endoscopic ulcers induced by NSAID/L-aspirin are associated with anemia, implying bleeding from ulcers.

Methods: This retrospective cohort study enrolled consecutive RA outpatients with a recorded medical history of >3 months to participate in this study at Nippon Medical School. These patients underwent esophagogastroduodenoscopy (EGD). Subjects receiving proton pump inhibitors or prostaglandin E1 analog co-therapy or who displayed any changes in medication within the preceding 3 months were excluded from this investigation. Patients were then divided into 4 groups according to the pattern of NSAID/L-aspirin administration: controls (n=25); NSAID group (n=174); NSAID+Aspirin group (n=11); and NSAID+NSAID group (n=22). Hemoglobin level (Hb) and mean corpuscular volume (MCV) were used as biomarkers for potential bleeding.

Results: Ulcer incidence was 0% in the control group, 19.5% in the NSAID group, 18.2% in the NSAID+aspirin group, and 45.5% in the NSAID+NSAID group. Ulcer incidence was higher in the NSAID group than in the control group (P=0.010), and ulcer incidence was higher in the NSAID+NSAID group than in the control or NSAID groups (P=0.010 and P=0.012, respectively).

Conversely, no significant differences were seen in biomarkers (Hb or MCV) for potential bleeding among the four groups. To clarify the association of endoscopic peptic ulcers with potential bleeding, each group was divided into two subgroups: with endoscopic peptic ulcer, and without endoscopic peptic ulcer. In subgroups with endoscopic peptic ulcer, Hb was lower in the NSAID+aspirin group than in the NSAID group or NSAID+NSAID group (P=0.010 and P=0.010, respectively).

Furthermore, in the NSAID+aspirin group, Hb in the subgroup with endoscopic peptic ulcer tended to be low compared to that in the subgroup without endoscopic peptic ulcer (P=0.055), and MCV was significantly lower in the subgroup with endoscopic peptic ulcer than in the subgroup without endoscopic peptic ulcer (P=0.029).

Conclusions: Non-aspirin NSAID-duplicated therapy has a higher risk of peptic ulcer compared with NSAID alone, but L-aspirin-NSAID combination therapy does not. Nevertheless, endoscopic ulcers with combined NSAID/L-aspirin therapy, but not in the other groups, seem to have a risk of potential bleeding, even if the ulcers are asymptomatic.

Chapter 4 – Background: Studies on the effects of gender and smoking on cardiovascular and peptic ulcer disease have been reported in Western countries, but data from Asian countries are limited and inconsistent.

Methods: The authors examined the effects of gender and smoking on cardiovascular and peptic ulcer disease using the longitudinal data of the Adult Health Study collected during biennial health examinations from 1 July 1958 to 30 June 1998. The examinations included medical history, chest x-ray, ultrasonography, and fluoroscopy or endoscopy. Smoking histories were obtained from 5 questionnaires self-administered during different time periods. The authors estimated the relative risks for being female and for "ever" versus "never" smoking after adjusting for significant effects of age, city, birth cohort, calendar time, alcohol intake, and radiation dose. The authors also examined the interaction between gender and smoking.

Results: Eight hundred and fifty four strokes, 215 aortic aneurysms, 1093 gastric ulcers, and 437 duodenal ulcers were detected between 1958 to 1998: and, from 1978 to 1998, 125 myocardial infarction were detected. The incidence of myocardial infarction, stroke, and gastric and duodenal ulcer was significantly higher in men than in women, but the authors found no gender difference for aortic aneurysm incidence after adjustment for smoking status. The authors detected positive associations of smoking with myocardial infarction (RR for ever smoked to never smoked, 1.96), stroke (RR, 1.26), aortic aneurysm (RR, 1.80), gastric ulcer (RR, 2.06), and duodenal ulcer (RR, 1.32). The interaction between gender and smoking status was not significant for any of the diseases.

Conclusions: Male gender and smoking were significant risk factors for cardiovascular and peptic ulcer disease in a Japanese population.

Chapter 5 - Acute gastric mucosal lesions, which can develop within a few hours after polytrauma, shock, major operations, central nervous system lesions, or severe infection, cause about one third of the cases of gastrointestinal bleeding. The authors analyzed and compared the effectiveness of two antisecretory compounds such as cimetidine and omeprazole on acute gastric mucosal lesions and acidity induced by stress in rats. Male Sprague-Dawley rats after 24 h fasting, received omeprazole (2.9–29 μmol/kg p.o.), cimetidine (99–396 μmol/kg p.o.) or their respective vehicle 1 h before being exposed to water immersion stress for 3 h. All rats were ulcer-indexed according to the length and number of their ulcers.

The stomach contents were aspirated for acid output and pH analysis. Omeprazole was more effective than cimetidine in keeping gastric pH high and lowering the total gastric acid output. Macroscopical examination of acute gastric mucosal erosions showed that omeprazole was 10 times more effective than cimetidine on molar basis in the inhibition of ulcer formation. The sudden increase in pH afforded by proton pump inhibitors indicate them as first-line therapy for treatment and prophylaxis of stress ulcer patients.

Chapter 7 - Although it has been well established that opioid analgesics relieve pain by acting on receptors in the central nervous system, research has suggested that similar analgesia can be achieved through peripheral opioid receptors. Basic science research has demonstrated that malignant or benign skin ulcers can expose peripheral sensory nerve terminals, while local inflammation within the ulcer up-regulates opioid receptors. Thus, one strategy to manage pain arising from these ulcers would be to apply topical opioid agonists, usually in the form of a gel. While systemic absorption likely varies with extent of ulceration, topical analgesics could reduce the need for systemic medications and the resultant adverse effects. However, research in the area has been slow; a few small randomized trials and case series suggest benefits from morphine gel. Whether it is a placebo effect or actual analgesia produced from peripheral receptors, many unfortunate patients suffer from difficult to treat ulcerative pain and may appear to benefit from a topical strategy. Larger studies are needed and, fortunately, are being conducted to help establish topical opioid therapy as a viable adjunct to systemic therapy in treating pain from ulcers.

In: Ulcers: Causes, Diagnosis, and Treatment ISBN: 978-1-60741-253-3
Editors: Danijel Erceg et al. pp. 1-19

Chapter 1

PSYCHOSOCIAL DISTRESS AS A RISK FACTOR OF PEPTIC ULCER MORTALITY

Y. E. Razvodovsky*
Grodno State Medical University, Belarus.

INTRODUCTION

Peptic ulcer disease (PUD) is one of the common disorders affecting the digestive system. The lifetime risk of ulcer is 5–10% in developed countries [31]. The pathology of ulcer is complex and may involve overproduction of acid or pepsin, inadequate mucosal defense, or reflux of bile and pancreatitic juice into the stomach [28]. Peptic ulcer is a classical example of the biopsychosocial model of disease, and like most diseases, it has a multifactorial origin. Although Helicobacter pyloris is considered causal for ulcer, a variety of host factors besides infection may play an important contributing role for this disease: smoking, alcohol consumption, non-steroid anti-inflammatory drug use and psychosocial distress [8]. Peptic ulcer is a remarkable model for understanding the complex interactions between psychosocial, socioeconomic, behavioral and infection factors in the etiology of organic pathology.

* Corresponding Author: e-mail: razvodovsky@grsmu.by yury_razvodovsky@mail.ru

The relationship between stress and ulcer has been shown in a large series of methodologically sound studies. In his comprehensive review, Levenstein has argued that stress contributes to the etiology of between 30% and 65% of peptic ulcer cases [20]. Moreover, a recent update concluded that psychosocial stress is a major risk factor of ulcer, since Helicobacter is inadequate as a monocausal explanation, as most infected people do not develop ulcer. Several longitudinal follow-up studies have shown that psychological distress, self-described as "stress or strain", or concrete life stressors at baseline increase the risk of ulcer development over the next 9 to 15 years [15,17]. One longitudinal study based on data from the National Health and Nation Examination Survey (a nationally representative cohort study of US adults) showed that after adjustment for potential confounders (age, sex, education, smoking, and regular aspirin use) persons who perceived themselves as stressed were 1.8 times (95% confidence interval 1.3 to 2.5) more likely to develop ulcers than those who did not [1]. A greater relationship was found between the perceived amount of stress and the incidence of peptic ulcer: relative to nonstressed persons, the relative risk of developing an ulcer was 1.4, 1.9, 2.3, 2.4, and 2.9 at five increasing levels of stress. In another well-designed Alameda County Study, subjects with high levels of psychological distress had age-adjusted odds of 2.8 for developing an ulcer over the following 9 years, signifying an excess risk of 180% over the reference level of 1.0, which fell to 2.2 (120% excess risk) after adjustment for potential confounders [17]. A substantial body of empirical evidence suggests that collective disasters can provoke ulceration: the German blitz in London [32], the Kobe earthquake [3], the economic crisis in Sophia [25] have been followed by an increase of hospitalizations for perforated stomach and duodenum ulcer. Such stressors as unemployment, marital strain and children's problems were also associated with increased ulcer incidence [9,15,16].

Recent investigations have contributed evidence concerning the relationship between depression/anxiety and risk of PUD. The studies had shown that generalized anxiety disorder (GAD) was associated with an increased likelihood of self-reported PUD among adults in the general population [11]. Moreover, a dose-response relationship between PUD and GAD symptoms was established [11]. These findings are consistent with data from clinical settings suggesting that PUD occurs more frequently among individuals with anxiety and depressive disorders [16]. These data are especially relevant in the light of prospective clinical studies that have reported that psychological distress, depression and anxiety are associated with poorer gastric ulcer healing [12,20].

One of the most interesting aspects of worldwide health trends in the late-twentieth century was the fluctuation in mortality rate over time in Russia: decline between 1985 and 1987, followed by a dramatic increase in the early 1990s. Several scholars have argued that the psychosocial distress resulting from the dramatic social, economic and political changes have played a crucial role in the Russian mortality crisis in the early 1990s [10,30,34]. However, it is extremely difficult to test the causal relationship between psychosocial distress and mortality because there are no direct indicators of stress at the population level. Taking into account experimental and empirical evidence, we can assume that suicide rate may better capture the magnitude of psychosocial distress than factors usually referred to as hypothetical stressors, e.g., unemployment and inflation rates, family instability (divorces), labor turnover and income inequality. To test this hypothesis, trends in the suicide (as an integral indicator for psychosocial distress) and PUD mortality rate in Russia from 1965 to 2005 were analyzed employing ARIMA time series analysis.

Material and Methods

The data on age-adjusted sex-specific mortality rates per 1,000,000 residents were taken from the Russian vital statistics registration system. Concerning issues of data quality, earlier studies have confirmed the reliability of the vital statistics for the Soviet [37] and post Soviet period [33].

The research evidence suggests that up to 44% of the adverse effects of stress on PUD may be attributed to stress-associated behavior such as smoking and alcohol consumption [18]. In Russia the fatal alcohol poisoning rate is likely to be a good measure of heavy episodic drinking [26]. Therefore, the fatal alcohol poisoning rate was included in the analysis as an indicator of binge drinking. Data on cigarette sales were not presented in this study.

The statistical analysis was conducted with the package "Statistica". It is generally agreed that bivariate correlations between two raw time-series are spurious due to common sources of trends and autocorrelation [24]. Therefore in order to reduce the risk of obtaining a spurious relation between two variables that have common trends, the trends should be removed by means of differencing procedure: $\nabla x_t = x_t - x_{t-1}$ This means analyzing annual changes rather than raw data. The process of removing systematic variation within a time series prior to the examination of potential causal relationships is referred to as "prewhitening". The residuals of a statistically adequate time series are distributed as a white noise process. A further step entails the inspection of cross correlation function in order to estimate the association between the two prewhitened time series. The final step involves a number of diagnostic checks (calculating a Box-Jenkins test statistic for the null hypothesis in order to show that the model residuals are distributed as white noise, and a Box-Ljung Q-test statistic for the null hypothesis to demonstrate that the set of values for the cross correlations is jointly independent). This technique for undertaking a time series analysis was suggested by Box and Jenkins and is often referred to as the ARIMA (autoregressive integrated moving average) model [4]. We used this model to estimate the relationship between the time series of suicide (as a proxy for psychosocial distress) and PUD mortality rate in this paper. A change in aggregate level drinking is expected to have an immediate effect on acute forms of alcohol-related problems (such as accidents and injuries), as well as a long-term effect on chronic problems (liver cirrhosis). Since peptic ulcer attributed to the chronic rather than acute alcohol-related problems, we should expect that the mortality response to changes in aggregate level alcohol consumption will be distributed over several years. Thus, we should consider the time-lag problem. In order to deal with this problem we inspected the cross-correlations between the time series at different lags.

Results

According to official statistics, the PUD mortality rate increased 2.4 times (from 17.7 to 41.7 per 1,000,000 residents) for males and 4.7 times (from 2.6 to 12.3 per 1000.000 of residents) for females in Russia from 1965 to 2005. The fatal alcohol poisoning rate for males increased 2.9 times (from 159.7 to 468.7 per 1,000,000 population), and for females increased 4.1 times (from 27.9 to 113.6 per 1,000,000 of population). The suicide rate for males increased by 33.8% (from 447.5 to 598.8 per 1,000,000 population), while the rate for females decreased by 7.3% (from 101.0 to 93.7 per 1,000,000 population). It should be noted that the male PUD mortality rate was significantly higher than the female rate with a ratio of 5.5 in 1965 decreasing to 2.4 by 2005. The trends in age-adjusted, sex-specific mortality rates are displayed in Figures 1–4. As can be seen, suicide, alcohol poisoning and PUD mortality rates for males seem to follow each other across the 1965–2005 time series. The time series fluctuated over the period: increased steadily from 1965 to 1980, then dropped sharply in the mid-1980s and dramatically jumped in the early 1990s.

Table 1. Cross-correlation function: male suicide rate (independent variable) and PUD mortality rate (dependent variable).

Lag	r	S.E.
-5	-0.138	0.224
-4	-0.239	0.218
-3	-0.269	0.213
-2	-0.120	0.209
-1	0.448	0.204
0	0.791	0.200
1	0.415	0.204
2	-0.022	0.209
3	-0.161	0.213
4	0.200	0.218
5	0.059	0.224

Table 2. Cross-correlation function: male fatal alcohol poisoning rate (independent variable) and PUD mortality rate (dependent variable).

Lag	r	S.E.
-5	-0.005	0.167
-4	-0.006	0.164
-3	-0.043	0.162
-2	-0.016	0.160
-1	-0.052	0.158
0	0.147	0.160
1	0.485	0.162
2	0.363	0.164
3	-0.105	0.164
4	-0.206	0.164
5	-0.374	0.169

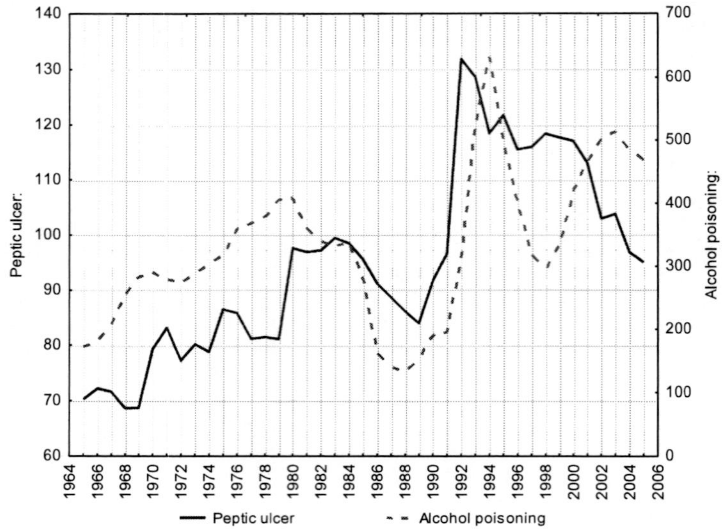

Figure 1. Trends in PUD and alcohol poisoning mortality rates for males in Russia from 1965 to 2005.

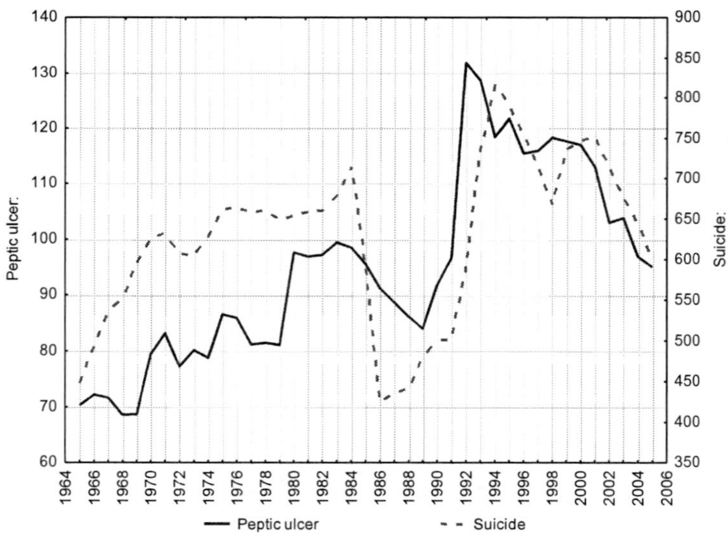

Figure 2. Trends in PUD and suicide mortality rates for males in Russia from 1965 to 2005.

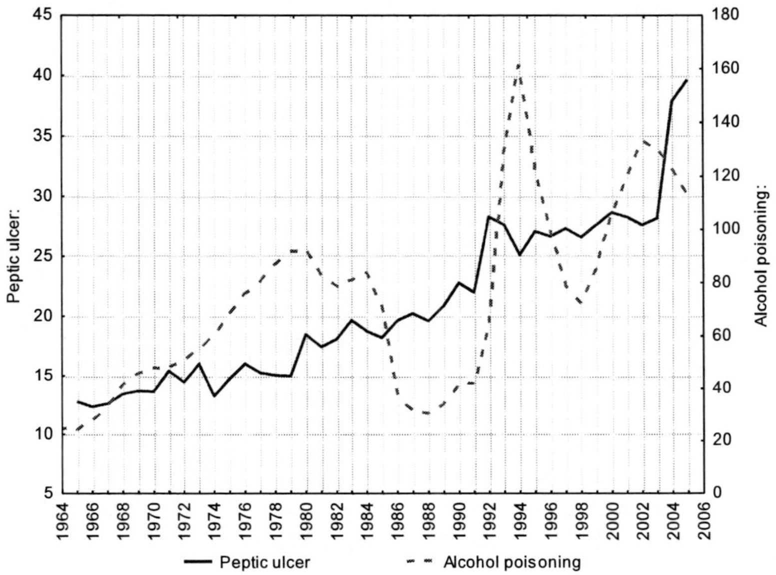

Figure 3. Trends in PUD and alcohol poisoning mortality rates for females in Russia from 1965 to 2005.

Table 3. Cross-correlation function: female suicide rate (independent variable) and PUD mortality rate (dependent variable).

Lag	r	S.E.
-5	0.139	0.169
-4	-0.258	0.167
-3	-0.093	0.164
-2	0.097	0.162
-1	-0.289	0.160
0	-0.006	0.158
1	-0.037	0.160
2	0.069	0.162
3	0.107	0.164
4	0.031	0.167
5	-0.141	0.169

It is important to point out that the pattern male and female suicide and fatal alcohol poisoning rates is quite similar over time, while there is a substantial difference between the sex-specific PUD mortality trends. For instance, the upward trend in PUD mortality rate across the time series has been greater for women than for men. Further, the decrease in PUD mortality rate in the mid-1980s and the subsequent increase in the early 1990s was substantially greater for men: between 1984 and 1989 the male rate decreased by 14.7%, while the female rate decreased by 7.4% from 1983 and 1985. Similarly, the male ulcer mortality rate increased by 57% from 1989 to 1992 and the female rate increased by 36.1%. Thus, the male PUD mortality rate tends to fluctuate across time series to a much greater extent than the female rate.

A Spearman's correlation analysis suggests quite a strong association between the suicide and PUD mortality ($r = 0.67$; $p = 0.000$), and between alcohol poisoning and PUD mortality ($r = 0.61$; $p = 0.000$) for males. The association between the suicide and PUD mortality ($r = 0.47$; $p = 0.002$) and between alcohol poisoning and PUD mortality ($r = 0.92$; $p = 0.000$) for females was also positive and statistically significant.

As can be seen from Figures 1–4, there are linear and S-shape trends in the time series. These trends were removed by means of a first-order differencing and specification as a first order moving average parameter (figures 5–6). After pre-whitening the cross-correlations between suicide, fatal alcohol poisoning and PUD, mortality time series were inspected. The outcome indicated a statistically significant cross-correlation between the suicide and PUD mortality rates for males at zero lag ($r = 0.75$; $SE = 0.20$) and at first lag ($r = 0.42$; $SE = 0.20$)(table 1). There is also positive cross-correlation between alcohol poisoning and PUD rates for men at first lag ($r = 0.49$; $SE = 0.16$) and at second lag ($r = 0.36$; $SE = 0.16$)(table 2).

The cross-correlation between alcohol poisoning and PUD for women is also positive, however, statistically not significant (table 3). At the same time, there is no cross-correlation between suicide and PU mortality for females (table. 4). So, positive correlation between these variables was spurious. The specification of the bivariate ARIMA model and outcome of the analyses are presented in Table 5. It can be seen, that the estimated effects of suicide on PUD mortality for males are clearly statistically significant. The estimated effects of fatal alcohol poisoning on PUD mortality for males are below statistical significance.

Discussion

Before considering the implications of this study, it is necessary to discuss alcohol policy issues. Alcohol control policies in Russia have undergone dramatic changes in the second half of the 20th century, ranging from tough restrictions in the mid 1980s, to an absolute lack of control following the collapse of the Soviet Union in 1991. In 1972 a resolution by the CPSU Central Committee "About the Measures Restricting Alcohol Consumption" was passed. According to the document, the production of vodka and the number of shops selling it were to be cut. There was evidence that anti-alcohol measures did lead to a slight decrease in alcohol-related mortality rate [22]. In 1973 a network of "commissions for the struggle against alcoholism" was established and from 1976 a narcological service began to operate. The beginning of the 1980s was marked by a new attempt to fight alcohol-related problems. The new Soviet leaders, Andropov first and then Chernenko, took a number of measures aimed at alcohol availability restriction. It was done within a campaign to strengthen public order and discipline in the workplace. There was evidence that official politics taken resulted in a decline of both alcohol consumption per capita and alcohol-related mortality levels [22].

In May 1985 M. Gorbachev launched the anti-alcohol campaign in response to high level of alcohol consumption and alcohol-related problems. The campaign restricted hours of alcohol sales, increased the price of alcohol, implemented purchase quotas, imposed tougher legal sanctions on home production and destroyed most of the vineyards across a number of Soviet republics. However, despite these efforts anti-alcohol campaign failed dramatically because the severe restrictions brought to the fore rapid grows of home brewing and substantial improvement in alcohol-related phenomena following the campaign was short-lived [23]. Major social, political and economic changes throughout the 1990s caused dramatic grows in alcohol consumption. Increasing alcohol consumption was one of the outcomes of collapse following "shock therapy" economic reforms that left a majority of the population below poverty level. In June 1992 the state alcohol monopoly was abolished as part of the economic liberalization that lead to the fragmentation of the alcohol industry. The country was practically flooded by a wave of homemade, counterfeit, and imported alcohol of low quality. The negative outcomes during transitional period included a sharp rise in alcohol-related mortality [22,23]. Over the recent years, the alcohol market became better controlled by the government; as a consequence, alcohol-related mortality rate was substantially reduced [23].

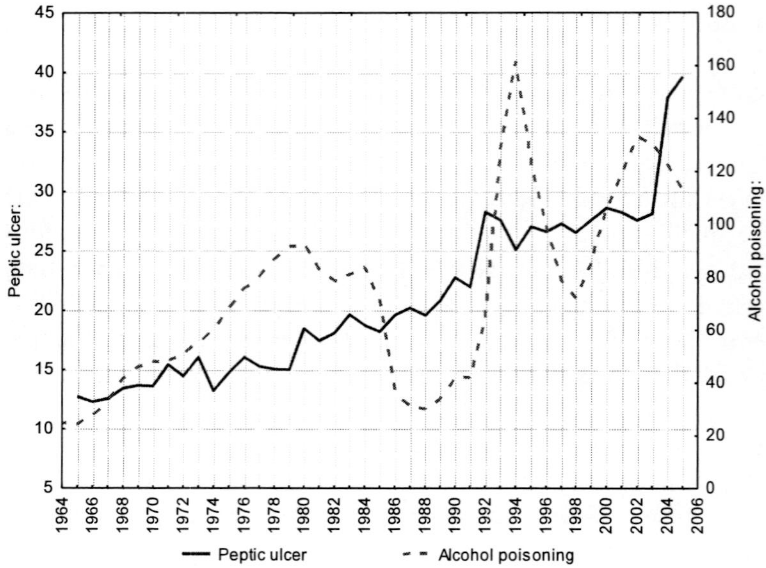

Figure 3. Trends in PUD and alcohol poisoning mortality rates for females in Russia from 1965 to 2005.

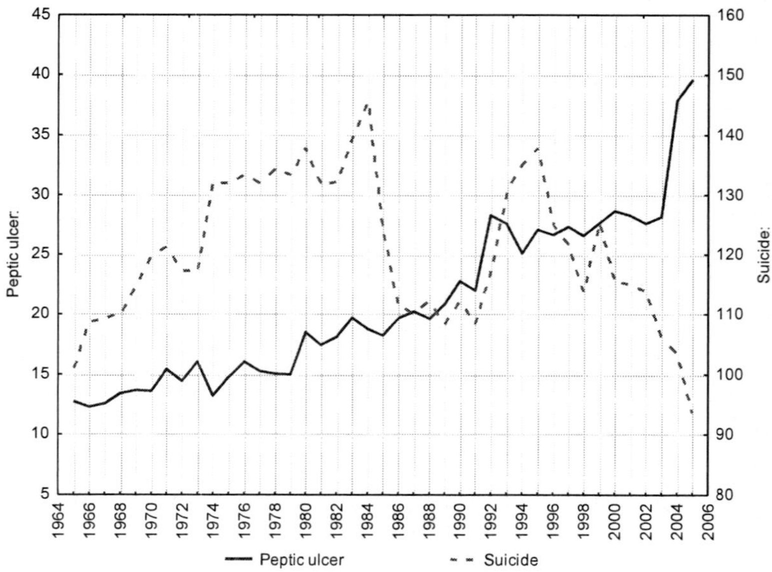

Figure 4. Trends in PUD and suicide mortality rates for males in Russia from 1965 to 2005.

The experience of Russia during the last decades presents a remarkable opportunity to examine the role of psychosocial factors in the etiology of organic pathology. As can be seen, the mortality trends have been more or less correlated with the great societal transformation. The substantial decreases in the time series in the mid-1980s corresponds with the anti-alcohol campaign of 1985-1988, witch significantly reduced alcohol consumption by limiting its manufacture and availability, and the dramatic increases in the early 1990s corresponds with the profound socio-economic and political changes occurring during the transitional period to the post communism. It also seems plausible, that suicide, alcohol poisoning and PUD mortality rates increase observed in the yearly 1990s resulted from the socio-economic crisis and anomic conditions was reinforced by the abolishing the state alcohol monopoly in 1992. The shock in the early 1990s was followed by a period of relative improvement and stability in the middle years of the decade. The subsequent rise in the suicide and alcohol poisoning rates from 1998 may be associated with the financial crisis and a worsening economic situation.

Table 4. Cross-correlation function: female fatal alcohol poisoning rate (independent variable) and PUD mortality rate (dependent variable).

Lag	r	S.E.
-5	0.069	0.169
-4	0.031	0.167
-3	0.105	0.164
-2	0.096	0.162
-1	-0.170	0.160
0	-0.139	0.158
1	0.211	0.160
2	0.203	0.162
3	-0.081	0.164
4	0.023	0.167
5	-0.167	0.169

Table 5. Estimated effects (bivariate ARIMA model) of suicide on male PUD mortality.

		Estimates	Std Error	t	Approx Sig
Non-Seasonal Lags	MA1	0,312	0,161	1,943	,050
Regression Coefficients		0,822	0,188	4,350	,000
Constant		0,010	0,004	2,423	,021

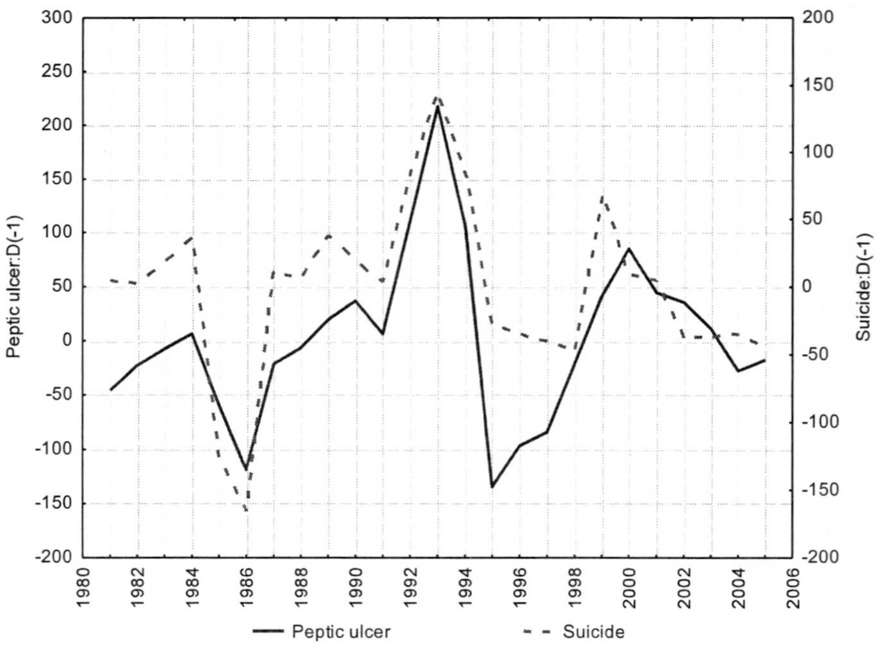

Figure 5. Trends PUD and suicide rates for males in Russia between 1980 and 2005 after differencing procedure.

The results from the time series analysis suggest a positive relationship between suicide (as a proxy for psychosocial distress) and PUD mortality for male at zero and at first lag. As a matter of fact the almost contemporaneous association between the two variables may support the point that psychosocial distress is a risk factor for peptic ulcer death. Moreover, the dynamics in suicide and PUD mortality rates for male in the 1990s fits a typical stress-related pattern: dramatic growth in the early 1990s (the acute stage) and decrease in the late 1990s (the stage of adaptation). This empirical evidence supports the concept of male depressive syndrome. This syndrome comprises low stress-tolerance, acting-out behavior, low impulse-control, substance abuse and a hereditary loading of depressive illness, alcoholism and suicide [36].

Here we should discuss the potential limitations of this study that may have affected the outcome. One can assume that the suicide and PUD mortality trends are being influenced by a confounding variable i.e. that the correlation is spurious. Most experts agree that the alcohol plays a significant role in decrease of mortality rates in the mid 1980s and subsequent dramatic grows in the early 1990s [14,22,23,33]. Other words, alcohol may be an important underlying factor of the fluctuation both suicide and ulcer mortality rates in Russia during the last decades. There is large body of clinical and research evidence that excessive alcohol consumption increase the risk of ulcer by impairing of the mucosal defense mechanisms [6,7,21]. In one longitudinal prospective study it was shown that, when compared with those who consumed less than 1.5 units of alcohol per week, individuals who consumed >63 units of alcohol per week 4 time more likely to develop bleeding ulcer [2]. On the other hand, several large-scale prospective studies have suggested a protective effect of moderate alcohol consumption (one or two drink a day) on the development of gastric ulcer [8,9]. In the prospective cohort study, a tendency towards an increase in the ulcer incidence proportion with the number of consumed drinks was observed resulting in a U-shaped relationship [29]. Several researchers reported protective effect of wine and beer consumption against the active Helicobacter pylori infection [5,9]. There are several possible biological mechanisms that could explain the protective effects of moderate alcohol consumption: 1) moderate alcohol intake might invigorate the mucosal defense by its effects on prostaglandins, 2) the increased gastrin secretion and resulting rise in gastric acid production enhance the antibacterial activity, 3) wine has a strong antibacterial effect [5,38]. There is also evidence of beverage-specific effect of alcohol on ulcer risk: wine drinking showed a protective effect against ulceration, whereas intake of spirits increased ulcer risk [27,29]. Studies that addressed the role of drinking pattern in relation to risk of ulcer suggest that binge drinking substantially increases the risk. For example, the Danish study provides evidence that wine drinking is associated with a much lower risk than beer drinking [2]. This might reflect the fact that beer drinkers are more likely to take alcohol in a binge session than wine drinkers. Thus, research evidence suggests that alcohol consumption may be related to positive or negative risk factors of ulcer, depending on the dose and type of drinking.

The results from the cross-correlation analysis suggest a positive relationship between fatal alcohol poisoning (as a proxy for binge drinking) and PUD mortality for males at first and second lags. Therefore, we have a reason to believe that, in this case, the independent variable is influencing the dependent variable, and that there is evidence of a lagged relationship between the two time series. It is important to point out that the size of the bivariate association between alcohol poisoning and ulcer for men is substantially greater than for women. It should be noted also that decreases in the two time series for males corresponds with the anti-alcohol campaign of 1985–1988. These facts are especially relevant in light of empirical evidence that suggests that in Russia binge drinking is a deeply rooted part of the male culture [22]. However, it seems plausible that alcohol is not a sufficient explanatory factor for the significant decrease in ulcer mortality rate in the mid 1980s. This phenomenon could have been related at least partially to the political and social liberalization during the period known as "perestroika" (1985–1990) [35]. Several researchers also believed that the increase in alcohol consumption in the 1990s was driven by the psychosocial distress of economic and political reforms [30,31]. The marked discrepancy between the two time series for males: upward trend of fatal alcohol poisoning and downward trend of ulcer mortality rate in 1998–2003 support stress-related hypothesis. So, rather than playing the major causal role, binge drinking may represent a confounding factor.

Another potential confounder of the stress-ulcer association is smoking. The research evidence suggests that tobacco smoking causes a significant increase in the risk of developing an ulcer [39]. Moreover, dose-response dependence was shown between the PUD risk and cumulative number of cigarettes [29]. Smoking more than 15 cigarettes per day raised the risk of perforated ulcer more than threefold as compared with lifetime abstinence from smoking [2]. Tobacco smoking seems to be an even more important risk factor for PUD than H. pylori infection [29]. It was shown that both gastric and ulcer disease were strongly associated with cigarette smoking, even after controlling for other potential risk factors [2]. The concurrent consumption of alcohol and cigarette smoking dose-dependently potentiated the ethanol-induced gastric mucosal damage [13]. The reduction of mucus secretion, increase in leukotriene B1 concentration, myeloperoxidase and inducible nitric oxide synthase activities accompanied such potentiating effect [6]. The findings also suggest that chronic nicotine treatment intensifies stress-evoked gastric ulceration [39]. The high prevalence of smoking among Russian men probably explains a part of the high male ulcer mortality rate compared with female mortality rate. However, there is little evidence of rapid changes in smoking pattern among Russian men in the early 1990s that has translated into the dramatic growth of the ulcer mortality rate. Therefore, further research is necessary to quantify the contribution of binge drinking and smoking to the PUD mortality.

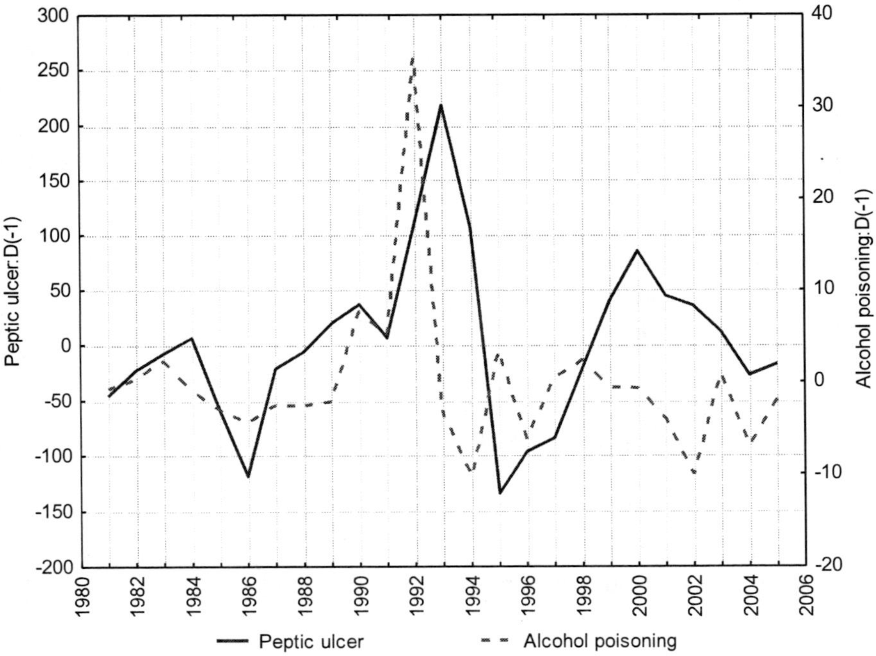

Figure 6. Trends in PUD and fatal alcohol poisoning rates for males in Russia between 1980 and 2005 after differencing procedure.

In conclusion, the results of the present study suggest a positive association between male suicide and peptic ulcer mortality rate at the aggregate level and support the hypothesis that psychosocial distress is a risk factor of ulcer at the individual level. Stress via direct pathophysiological mechanisms or through traditional risk factors (smoking, alcohol abuse) is linked to an increase of the ulcer mortality rate. The outcome of this study also supports the hypothesis that psychosocial distress, resulting from dramatic social, economic and political changes, has played an important role in the Russian mortality crisis in the early 1990s.

References

[1] Anda, RF; Williamson, DF; Escobedo, LG; Self-perceived stress and the risk of peptic ulcer disease. A longitudinal study of US adults. *Arch Intern Med,* 1992, 152, 829-33.

[2] Andersen, IB; Jørgensen T; Bonnevie, O; Smoking and alcohol intake as risk factors for bleeding and perforated peptic ulcers: a population-based cohort study. *Epidemiology,* 2000, 11, 434-9.

[3] Aoyama, N; Kinoshita, Y; Fujimoto, S; Himeno, S; Todo, A; Kasuga, M; Chiba, T. Peptic ulcers after the Hanshin-Awaji earthquake: increased incidence of bleeding gastric ulcers. *Am J Gastroenterol,* 1998; 93, 311-6.

[4] Box, GEP; Jenkins, GM. *Time Series Analysis: forecasting and control.* London. Holden-Day Inc., 1976

[5] Brenner, H; Rothenbacher, D; Bode, G. Inverse graded relation between alcohol consumption and active infection with Helicobacter pylori. *Am J Epidemiol*, 1999, 149, 571-6.

[6] Chou, SP. An examination of the alcohol consumption and peptic ulcer association—Results of a national survey. *Alcohol Clin Exp Res*, 1994, 18, 149-53.

[7] Chow, jY; Ma, L; Zhu, M; Cho, CH. The potentiating actions of cigarette smoking on ethanol-induced gastric mucosal damage in rats. *Gastroenterology*, 1997, 113(4), 1188-97.

[8] Everhart, JE; Kruszon-Moran, D; Perez-Peres, GI; Seroprevalence and ethnic differences in Helicobacter pylori infection among adults in the Unites States. *J Infect Dis,* 2000, 181, 1359-63.

[9] Everhart, JE; Byrd-Holt, D; Sonnenberg, A. Incidence and risk factors for self-reported peptic ulcer disease in the United States. *Am J Epidemio*, 1998, 147, 529-36.

[10] Gavrilova, NS., Semyonova, VG; Evdokushkina, GN; Gavrilov, LA. The response of violent mortality to economic crisis in Russia. *Population Research and Policy Review,* 2000, 19, 397-419.

[11] Goodvin, RD; Murray, BS. Generalized anxiety disorder and peptic ulcer disease among adults in the US. *Psychosomatic Medicine*, 2002, 64, 862-866.

[12] Holtmann, G; Armstrong, D; Pöppel, E; Bauerfeind, A; Goebell, H; Arnold, R; Classen, M; Witzel, L; Fischer, M; Heinisch, M; Blum, AL; members of the RUDER Study Group. Influence of stress on the healing and relapse of duodenal ulcers. *Scand J Gastroenterol,* 1992, 27, 917-23.

[13] Ko, JK; Cho, CH. Alcohol drinking and cigarette smoking: a "partner" for gastric ulceration. *Zhonghua Yi Xue Za Zhi,* 2000, 63(12), 845-54.

[14] Leon, DA; Chenet, L; Shkolnicov, VM. Huge variation in Russian mortality rates 1984-94: artefact, alcohol, or what? *Lancet*, 1997, 359, 383-388.

[15] Levenstein, S; Kaplan, GA; Smith, M. Sociodemographic characteristics, life stressors, and peptic ulcer: a prospective study. *J Clin Gastroenterol,* 1995, 21, 185-92

[16] Levenstein, S; Prantera, C; Scribano, ML; Varvo, V; Berto, E; Spinella, S. Psychologic predictors of duodenal ulcer healing. *J Clin Gastroenterol,* 1996, 22, 84-9.

[17] Levenstein, S; Kaplan, GA; Smith, MW. Psychological predictors of peptic ulcer incidence in the Alameda County Study. *J Clin Gastroenterol,* 1997, 24, 140-6.

[18] Levenstein, S. Stress and peptic ulcer: life beyond helicobacter. *BMJ*, 1998, 316, 538-41.

[19] Levenstein, S; Ackerman, S; Kiecolt-Glaser, JK; Dubols, A. Stress and peptic ulcer disease. *JAMA*, 1999, 281, 10-11.

[20] Levenstein, S. The very model of a modern etiology: a biopsychosocial view of peptic ulcer. *Psychosomatic Medicine,* 2000, 2, 176-185.

[21] Marotta, RB; Floch, MH. Diet and nutrition in ulcer disease. *Med Clin North Am,* 1991, 74, 967-79.

[22] Nemtsov, AV. *Alcohol related mortality in Russia*, 1980-90s., Moscow. 2001. Nalex.

[23] Nemtsov, AV; Razvodovsky, YE. Alcohol situation in Russia, 1980-2005. *Social and Clinical Psychiatry*, 2008, 2, 52-60.

[24] Norstrom, T; Skog, OJ. Alcohol and mortality: methodological and analytical issue in aggregate analysis. *Addiction,* 2001, 96, 5-17.

[25] Pomakov, P; Gueorgieva, S; Stantcheva, J; Tenev, T; Rizov, A. Ulcères gastro-duodenaux pendant la periode d'une crise economique aigue [Gastroduodenal ulcers during a period of acute economic crisis]. *J Radiol,* 1993, 74, 265–7.

[26] Pridemore, WA. Heavy drinking and suicide in Russia. *Social Forces,* 2006, 85(1), 413-430.

[27] Razvodovsky, YE. Aggregate level association between alcohol and the peptic ulcer mortality rate. *Alcoholism.*, 2006, 42(2), 61-68.

[28] Richardson, CT. Role of aggressive factors in the pathogenesis of peptic ulcer disease. *Scand J Gastroenterol*, 1990, 174(suppl), 37-43.

[29] Rosenstock, SJ; Jørgensen, T; Bonnevie O; Andersen, L. Risk factors for peptic ulcer disease: a population based prospective cohort study comprising 2416 Danish adults. *Gut*, 2003, 52, 186-193.

[30] Shkolnicov, VM.; Cornia, GA.; Leon, DA.; Mesle, F. Causes of the Russian mortality crisis: evidence and interpretations. *World Development*, 1998, 26, 1995-2011.

[31] Sonnenberg, A; Everhart, JE. Prevalence of self-reported peptic ulcer in the United States. *Am J Public Health,* 1996, 86, 200-5.

[32] Spicer CC; Stewart DN; Winser DMR. Perforated peptic ulcer during the period of heavy air raids. *Lancet,* 1944;1:14.

[33] Stickley, A; Leinsalu, M; Andreev, E; Razvodovsky, YE; Vagero, D; McKee, M. Alcohol poisoning in Russia and the countries in the European part of the former Soviet Union, 1970-2002. *European Journal of Public Health*, 2007, 17(5):444-449.

[34] Stone, R. Stress: The invisible hand in Eastern Europe's death rates. *Science,* 2000, 288, 1732-1733.

[35] Varnik, A; Wasserman, D; Dankowixz, M; Eklund, G. Age-specific suicide rates in the Slavic and Baltic regions of the former USSR during perestroika, in comparison with 22 European countries. *Acta Psychiatr Scand,* 1998, 98 (Suppl. 394), 20-25.

[36] Walinder L; Rutzt W. Male depression and suicide. *Int. Clin. Psychopharmacol,* 2001, 16(20), 21-4.

[37] Wasserman, D.; Varnik, A. Reliability of statistics on violent death and suicide in the former USSR, 1970-1990. *Acta Psychiatrica Scandinavica*, 1998, 394(Supplement), 34-41.

[38] Weisse, ME; Eberly, B; Person, DA. Wine as a digestive acid: comparative antimicrobial effects of bismuth salicylate and red and white wine. *BMJ*, 1995, 311, 1657-60.

[39] Wong, D; Koo, MW; Shin, VY. Pathogenesis of nicotine treatment and its withdrawal on stress-induced gastric ulceration in rats. *Eur J Pharmacol,* 2002, 34(1-2), 81-86.

In: Ulcers: Causes, Diagnosis, and Treatment ISBN: 978-1-60741-253-3
Editors: Danijel Erceg et al. pp. 21-36

Chapter 2

PEPTIC ULCER ASSOCIATED WITH NON-STEROIDAL ANTI-INFLAMMATORY DRUGS/LOW-DOSE ASPIRIN

Kazumasa Miyake**, *Taro Yoshioka, Hiroshi Nakamura and Choitsu Sakamoto,

[1]Department of Internal Medicine, Division of Gastroenterology, Nippon Medical School, Tokyo, Japan

[2]Department of Joint Disease and Rheumatism, Nippon Medical School, Tokyo, Japan

PURPOSE

Use of multiple non-steroidal anti-inflammatory drugs (NSAIDs) represents one of the risk factors for NSAID-associated peptic ulcer. However, insufficient evidence has been accumulated to conclude whether the risk of peptic ulcer increases with concomitant use of low-dose aspirin (L-aspirin) in long-term treatment with NSAID.

The majority of patients with rheumatoid arthritis (RA) display some of the risk factors for peptic ulcer and its complications. In addition, since long-term NSAID users, particularly RA patients, have a high risk of cardiovascular disease (CVD), determining the risk of peptic ulcer

* Corresponding Author: 1-1-5, Sendagi, Bunkyo-ku, Tokyo 113-8603, JAPAN, Tel: +81-3-3822-2131 Fax: +81-3-5685-1793, E-mail: km366@nms.ac.jp

induced by NSAID alone or in combination with L-aspirin in the daily clinical setting of RA patients is essential. The primary objective of this study was to elucidate the risk of peptic ulcer induced by concomitant L-aspirin in Japanese RA outpatients on long-term NSAID treatment. Although endoscopic ulcer has been defined as an excavated mucosal break ≥3 mm in diameter in most studies, the clinical implications of endoscopic ulcers are unclear. A secondary objective was thus to evaluate whether endoscopic ulcers induced by NSAID/L-aspirin are associated with anemia, implying bleeding from ulcers.

Methods

This retrospective cohort study enrolled consecutive RA outpatients with a recorded medical history of >3 months to participate in this study at Nippon Medical School. These patients underwent esophagogastroduodenoscopy (EGD). Subjects receiving proton pump inhibitors or prostaglandin E1 analog co-therapy or who displayed any changes in medication within the preceding 3 months were excluded from this investigation. Patients were then divided into 4 groups according to the pattern of NSAID/L-aspirin administration: controls (n=25); NSAID group (n=174); NSAID+Aspirin group (n=11); and NSAID+NSAID group (n=22). Hemoglobin level (Hb) and mean corpuscular volume (MCV) were used as biomarkers for potential bleeding.

Results

Ulcer incidence was 0% in the control group, 19.5% in the NSAID group, 18.2% in the NSAID+aspirin group, and 45.5% in the NSAID+NSAID group. Ulcer incidence was higher in the NSAID group than in the control group (P=0.010), and ulcer incidence was higher in the NSAID+NSAID group than in the control or NSAID groups (P=0.010 and P=0.012, respectively).

Conversely, no significant differences were seen in biomarkers (Hb or MCV) for potential bleeding among the four groups. To clarify the association of endoscopic peptic ulcers with potential bleeding, each group was divided into two subgroups: with endoscopic peptic ulcer, and without endoscopic peptic ulcer. In subgroups with endoscopic peptic ulcer, Hb was lower in the NSAID+aspirin group than in the NSAID group or NSAID+NSAID group (P=0.010 and P=0.010, respectively).

Furthermore, in the NSAID+aspirin group, Hb in the subgroup with endoscopic peptic ulcer tended to be low compared to that in the subgroup without endoscopic peptic ulcer (P=0.055), and MCV was significantly lower in the subgroup with endoscopic peptic ulcer than in the subgroup without endoscopic peptic ulcer (P=0.029).

Conclusions

Non-aspirin NSAID-duplicated therapy has a higher risk of peptic ulcer compared with NSAID alone, but L-aspirin-NSAID combination therapy does not. Nevertheless, endoscopic ulcers with combined NSAID/L-aspirin therapy, but not in the other groups, seem to have a risk of potential bleeding, even if the ulcers are asymptomatic.

INTRODUCTION

Non-steroidal anti-inflammatory drugs (NSAIDs) cause various mucosal injuries of the gastrointestinal tract, from asymptomatic endoscopic erosions/ulcers to ulcer accompanied by complications (mainly hemorrhage). As NSAIDs are one of the most widely used classes of drugs, ulcer hemorrhage requiring hospitalization has become an important consideration in Western countries. Conversely, with the increasing aging of society, the use of low-dose aspirin (L-aspirin) has spread rapidly as secondary prophylaxis against cardiovascular disease (CVD)[1]. Since L-aspirin results in both mucosal toxicity through cyclooxygenase (COX) and antiplatelet effects, the likelihood of an increase in peptic ulcers or associated complication remains a matter of concern.

However, insufficient evidence has been accumulated to conclude whether risk of peptic ulcer is increased with concomitant L-aspirin use during long-term treatment with NSAIDs. Overlapping use of NSAIDs and antiplatelet drugs is among the risk factors for NSAID ulcer complication to have already been indicated. Combined therapy with NSAID+L-aspirin is thought to increase the risk of peptic ulcer hemorrhage compared with NSAID alone or L-aspirin alone [1,2] Patients with rheumatoid arthritis (RA) often require long-term NSAID use, and also show several risk factors for peptic ulcer complications. In addition, risk of CVD and mortality in chronic-inflammation diseases such as RA have been shown to be higher than those in the general population [1,2,3,4]. In 2008 the European League Against Rheumatism (EULAR), Solomon DH and others had reported that both RA disease relevant gene (RA activity) and CVD risk factors affect the development of the acute myocardial infarction (AMI) and the CVA in RA patients. Furthermore, RA patients with high levels of the RA disease-relevant gene in addition to general CVD risks display an increasing need for prophylactic treatment against CVD using L-aspirin as an antiplatelet therapy. The concern is thus that concomitant use of NSAID and L-aspirin (NSAID+L-aspirin) increases the risks of developing peptic ulcer and hemorrhage. However, the risk of developing peptic ulcers with concomitant use of L-aspirin among long-term NSAID users has not yet been examined sufficiently. As a result, among RA outpatients regularly attending our hospital, incidence of endoscopic peptic ulcers was examined in subjects with concomitant use of NSAID+L-aspirin. Furthermore, although this point is arguable, most endoscopic peptic ulcers defined as excavated mucosal break ≥3 mm with unequivocal depth until now have been asymptomatic. The clinical implications of endoscopic ulcers are unclear. The secondary objective of the study was thus to evaluate whether the presence of endoscopic ulcers induced by co-therapy using L-aspirin with NSAID is implicated in potential bleeding from ulcers.

METHODS

This retrospective cohort study enrolled consecutive RA outpatients with a recorded medical history extending ≥3 months to participate in this study at Nippon Medical School from February 2003 to March 2007. All patients provided written informed consent and underwent esophagogastroduo denoscopy (EGD). Subjects who had been receiving proton pump inhibitors (PPI) or prostaglandin E1 analogs (PGs) as co-therapy or who had received any changes in medication within 3 months were excluded from this paper. Paired rheumatologists and gastroenterologists then began a structured interview and retrospective review of patient medical records to gather all relevant information, including demographics, concomitant medication and laboratory data. Concomitant medications including NSAIDs, corticosteroids, anti-rheumatoid agents, anti-coagulants, PPIs, PGs, and histamine-H2 receptor antagonists (H2RAs) such as anti-ulcer agents, and duration, frequency and dosage were collected for each medication. Eligible subjects included RA outpatients >20 years old with a history of ≥3 months on NSAID medication. Patients who had undergone stomach resections or *Helicobacter pylori* eradication therapy, had shown severe dyspeptic symptoms or gastrointestinal bleeding, or were pregnant or lactating were excluded from this study, along with patients who underwent changes to any of their prescriptions within the 3-month period prior to EGD, with the exception of NSAID medication. We did not exclude patients who, in addition to regular NSAID intake, were also on short-term (≤7 days) NSAID therapy for the treatment of acute conditions. Continuous users were defined as patients taking any medication for ≥4 days a week for a period of ≥3 months, irrespective of dosage. Warfarin and low-dose aspirin or any antiplatelet agents were defined as anti-coagulants. Patients were required to stop taking these drugs for a short period before endoscopy when possible. Patients were also questioned at the time of endoscopy regarding the presence or absence of four different dyspeptic symptoms: heartburn; epigastric pain; nausea/vomiting; and sensation of fullness. Symptoms were scored on 3 levels of severity: none, not present; mild, weak symptoms not requiring treatment; or severe, symptoms requiring treatment. Patients were then divided into 4 groups according to the pattern of taking NSAID/L-aspirin: controls (n=25); NSAID group (n=178); NSAID+aspirin group (n=11); and NSAID+NSAID group (n=19).

Hemoglobin level (Hb) and mean corpuscular volume (MCV) were used as biomarkers for potential bleeding.

This study was conducted in accordance with the guidelines of the Declaration of Helsinki.

Evaluation by Endoscopy

All RA outpatients who participated in this study underwent EGD to determine the presence or absence of any ulcers in the stomach or duodenum. Taking the phase of the healing cycle of ulcers into consideration, an ulcer was defined as an excavated mucosal break ≥3 mm in diameter with unequivocal depth measured using biopsy forceps. All endoscopic examinations were performed by three endoscopists and digitally recorded. Two experienced endoscopists who had each performed >2000 upper endoscopies were invited to assess these pictures, blinded to patient demographic data. We finally diagnosed mucosal breaks as endoscopic ulcer when both endoscopists agreed that a lesion represented an ulcer.

For each endoscopic examination, biopsy specimens from the antrum and corpus were obtained for histological analysis to determine the presence of *H. pylori*.

H. pylori infection

Based on the results of serologic tests for anti-*H. pylori* immunoglobulin G using an enzyme-linked immunosorbent assay (E-Plate, Eiken, Japan) and histological examination, *H. pylori* infection was diagnosed as positive when at least one of two tests showed positive results.

Statistical Analysis

Demographic and laboratory data were compared between groups, depending on the type of data analyzed, using the χ^2 test or Fisher's exact test for categorical data and unpaired Student's t-test for continuous variables.

We studied the incidence of dyspeptic symptoms by collecting data from a structured interview just prior to endoscopy. The association between peptic ulcer and dyspeptic symptoms was assessed using the χ^2 test. Differences with values of $p<0.05$ were regarded as statistically significant.

All statistical analyses were performed using SPSS software (SPSS, Chicago, IL).

RESULTS

We screened 256 patients by endoscopy between February 2003 and March 2007. Of these, 24 patients had undergone changes in the prescription of key drugs such as NSAIDs, corticosteroids, anti-rheumatoid agents, bisphosphonates, anti-coagulants and anti-ulcer drugs within 3 months prior to endoscopy.

In all, 232 RA outpatients (25 men, 207 women; mean age, 61.7 ±0.6 years) met our inclusion criteria and were included in this analysis. As baseline characteristics for all patients, mean duration of arthritis was 15.5 ±0.8 years and 35 patients (15.1%) had a past history of peptic ulcer disease. Corticosteroids had been used by 191 patients (82.4%), 190 patients (82.0%) had used anti-rheumatoid agents, 27 patients (11.6%), had used anti-coagulants and 111 patients (47.8%) displayed *H. pylori* infection.

Peptic ulcer was found in 46 of the 232 patients (19.8%), including 39 with gastric ulcer, 6 with duodenal ulcer, and 1 patient with both gastric and duodenal ulcers.

Table 1 compares demographic and laboratory data between the 4 groups categorized according to patterns of NSAID/L-aspirin use. Data on the following clinical parameters were analyzed: demographics of RA NSAID users including age, gender, disease duration; smoking; alcohol; history of peptic ulcer; *H. pylori* infection; and co-medication with drugs such as corticosteroids, anti-rheumatic agents, anti-coagulants and H2RAs. The percentage of anti-coagulant use was higher in the NSAID+Aspirin group than in any other group (P<0.01 each), but no other significant differences were seen among the three groups other than the NSAID+Aspirin group.

Table 1. Baseline characteristics in patients with rheumatoid arthritis

Characteristic	Control group (n=25)	NSAID group (n=174)	NSAID + Aspirin group (n=11)	NSAID + NSAID group (n=22)	*P value*
Age	60.1	61.5	64.0	64.4	NS
Female (%)	25 (100)	153 (87.9)	9 (81.8)	21 (95.5)	NS
Smoker (%)	3 (12.0)	35 (20.1)	1 (9.1)	6 (27.3)	NS
Alcohol (%)	5 (20.8)	47 (27.0)	2 (18.2)	4 (18.2)	NS
Duration of arthritis (years)	20.1	14.5	21.1	15.1	NS
Past history of PUD (%)	11 (47.8)	28 (16.3)	3 (27.3)	4 (18.2)	NS
Corticosteroids (%)	23 (92.0)	139 (79.9)	8 (72.7)	21 (95.5)	NS
Anti-rheumatic agents (%)	18 (72.0)	145 (83.3)	8 (72.7)	20 (90.9)	NS
Anti-coagulant agents (%)	* 1 (4.0)	* 14 (8.0)	<u>11 (100)</u>	* 1 (4.5)	$
H2 receptor antagonists (%)	8 (32.0)	52 (29.9)	4 (36.4)	11 (50.0)	NS
H. pylori infection (%)	11 (44.0)	85 (48.9)	5 (45.5)	10 (45.4)	NS
Dyspepsia (%)	10 (40.0)	90 (51.7)	5 (45.5)	10 (45.5)	NS

About half of all patients (49.6%) displayed mild dyspeptic symptoms. Epigastric pain was the most common of the four symptoms evaluated. Prevalence of dyspeptic symptoms showed no significant differences among groups.

Table 2. Biomarkers for potential bleeding in patients with rheumatoid arthritis

Group	n	Mean ±SE	
		Hb (g/dl)	MCV (fl)
Control	25	11.9 ±0.3	91.7 ±1.8
NSAID	174	12.2 ±0.1	92.7 ±1.1
NSAID +Aspirin	11	11.5 ±0.8	87.7 ±2.7
NSAID +NSAID	22	12.3 ±0.4	91.8 ±1.4

No significant differences between any groups

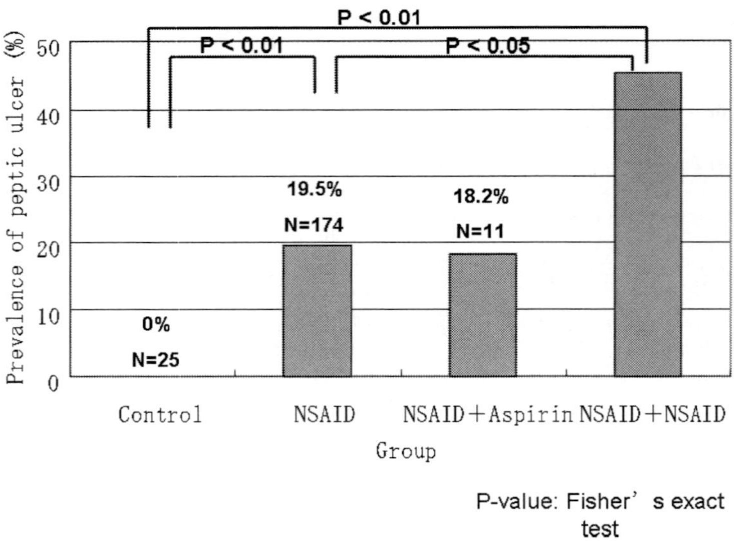

Figure 1. Prevalence of peptic ulcer in patients with rheumatoid arthritis

Ulcer incidence was 0% in the control group, 19.5% in the NSAID group, 18.2% in the NSAID+Aspirin group, and 45.5% in the NSAID+NSAID group (Figure 1). Ulcer incidence in the NSAID group was higher than that in the control group (P=0.010), and ulcer incidence was higher in the NSAID+NSAID group than in the control or NSAID groups (P=0.010 and P=0.012, respectively).

Table 3. Numbers in subgroups with and without peptic ulcers in patients with rheumatoid arthritis

		Subgroup with peptic ulcers	Subgroup without peptic ulcers
Control group	n=25	0	25
NSAID group	n=174	34	140
NSAID+Aspirin group	n=11	2	9
NSAID+NSAID group	n=22	10	12

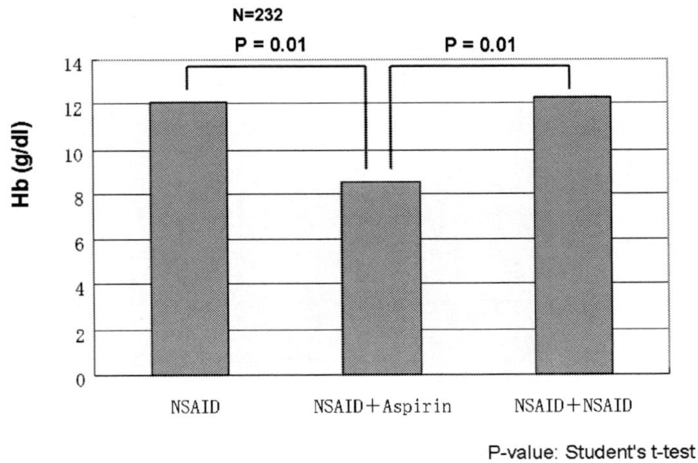

Figure 2. Hemoglobin levels in subgroup with peptic ulcers among patients with rheumatoid arthritis

On the other hand, no significant differences were seen in biomarkers (Hb, MCV) for potential bleeding among the four groups (Table 2). To clarify the association of endoscopic peptic ulcers with potential bleeding, each group was divided into two subgroups: with endoscopic peptic ulcer; and without endoscopic peptic ulcer (Table 3). In the subgroup with endoscopic peptic ulcer, Hb was lower in the NSAID+Aspirin group (8.5±1.5 g/dl) than in the NSAID group (12.1±0.3 g/dl) or NSAID+NSAID group(12.3±0.4 g/dl) (P=0.010 and P=0.010, respectively) (Figure 2).

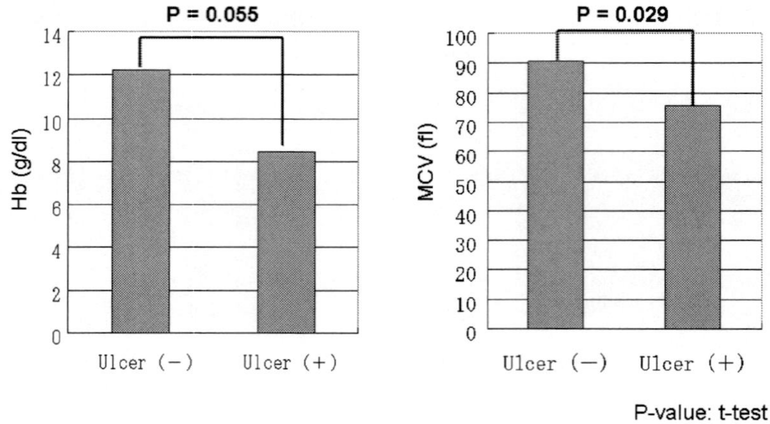

Figure 3. Hemoglobin and mean corpuscular erythrocyte volume between subgroups with and without peptic ulcers in the *NSAIDs + Aspirin* group

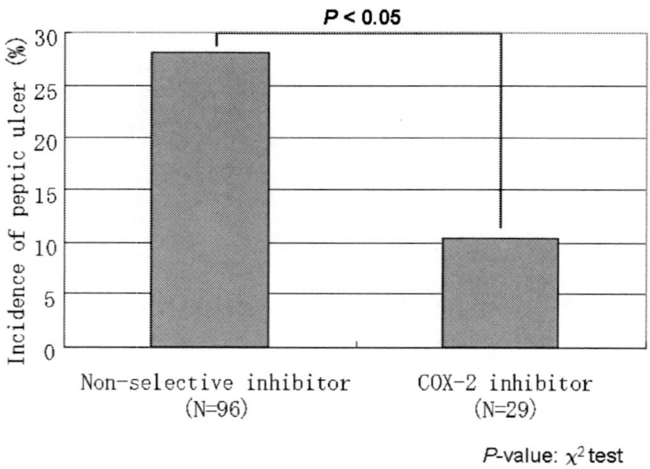

Figure 4. Incidence of peptic ulcer in single-NSAID-treated patients without anti-ulcer agents

Furthermore, in the NSAID+Aspirin group, Hb in the subgroup with endoscopic peptic ulcer tended to be low compared with that in the subgroup without endoscopic peptic ulcer (Hb: 8.5±1.5 g/dl vs. 12.2±0.73g/dl, P=0.055). MCV was significantly lower in the subgroup with endoscopic peptic ulcer than in the subgroup without endoscopic peptic ulcer (MCV: 75.8±2.5 fl vs. 90.4±2.5 fl; P=0.029) (Figure 3).

DISCUSSION

L-Aspirin and Mucosal Injuries

L-aspirin suppresses thromboxane (TX)A2 synthesis by irreversibly inhibiting cyclooxygenase (COX)-1 in platelets, and demonstrates a platelet aggregation-inhibiting action. L-aspirin is an antiplatelet drug that reduces the relapse of serious CVD resulting from atherothrombosis to about 25% [1,2]. In the guidelines of each country, antiplatelet therapy is mainly considered indispensable as secondary prophylaxis, and use of L-aspirin is thus increasing rapidly.

Although NSAID-associated upper gastrointestinal tract lesions vary, gastric mucosal injuries including erosion are seen commonly in ≥80% of NSAID users. In many endoscopic studies, the prevalence of peptic ulcer induced by conventional NSAIDs has been reported as 15–40% per year [1,2,3,4]. Conversely, peptic ulcer induced by L-aspirin has a reported incidence of around 28% per year, along with 11% prevalence and 1.2% bleeding rate [1,2]. However, since L-aspirin is a low-dose NSAID, the risks of gastroduodenal mucosal injuries by aspirin tend to have been underestimated in comparison to standard doses NSAID. The ulcer-hemorrhage rate by L-aspirin has not shown any dose-dependency in meta-analysis, and an equivalent hemorrhage risk even with low doses has been reported [1]. L-aspirin users have been shown to experience 7.7-times as many bleeding risks compared to the control in a multicenter case-control study from Japan, and this risk was considered equivalent or exceeding that of patients with "usual" NSAID doses (odds ratio, 7.3) [1]. Actually, the increasingly wide use of L-aspirin despite mucosal toxicity and antiplatelet effects has resulted in an increased prevalence of ulcer bleeding. Ulcer hemorrhage rate from L-aspirin use increased from 15 to 27 persons per 100,000 people from 1996 to 2002, although the ulcer hemorrhage rate associated with conventional NSAIDs decreased from 1996 to 2002 in Scotland with the appearance of specific COX-2 inhibitors [1].

Effects of COX-2 Selectivity on NSAID-Induced Mucosal Injuries

Differences in peptic ulcer development depending on the COX-2 selectivity of NSAID have been observed in many reports [1,2]. We conducted a subanalysis of the effects of COX-2 selectivity on endoscopic ulcer incidence. This subanalysis was conducted on 125 patients receiving NSAIDs for ≥3 months, excluding those receiving H2RAs, as well as PPI and prostaglandin E1 analogs demonstrating protective effects against peptic ulcer formation. Ulcer prevalence in 96 patients who received non-selective NSAIDs (loxoprofen, n=38; lornxicam, n=30; diclofenac, n=9; and one of five other drugs, n=19) and 29 patients who received etodolac, the main COX-2 inhibitor administered in this study, was 28.1% (27 patients) and 10.3% (3 patients), respectively. Ulcer incidence was significantly lower for COX-2 inhibitors (Figure 4; $P<0.05$). COX-2 inhibitors include those found as compounds causing fewer gastrointestinal events with gastrointestinal injury as the indicator, and those developed as compounds sparing gastrointestinal events by structural analysis of COX-2. Etodolac, which was placed in the COX-2 inhibitor group for this subanalysis, is included in the former, while coxibs such as celecoxib and rofecoxib are included in the latter. Specific COX-2 inhibitors such as celecoxib and rofecoxib had not been approved in Japan until just before the completion of this study. In the United States, etodolac, a COX-2 inhibitor (≥800 mg/day) or the non-selective NSAID naproxen (≥1000 mg/day) was administered without concomitant ulcer-inducing drugs excluding L-aspirin to 16,286 elderly patients. After examining upper gastrointestinal events, the incidence of upper gastrointestinal events was reported to be significantly lower in the etodolac group than in the naproxen group [1]. Our results prove that etodolac reduces ulcer incidence more than non-selective NSAIDs also in Japanese. COX-2 inhibitors are thus preferable in patients with high risk of ulcer development, such as elderly patients and patients with a history of ulcer.

Risk of Peptic Ulcer Induced by Concomitant L-Aspirin in Long-Term NSAID Treatment

Since L-aspirin therapy mainly inhibits intramucosal COX-1, concomitant use of NSAIDs is thought to increase the risk of ulcer hemorrhage regardless of any dosage or types of NSAIDs used together. Even if specific COX-2 inhibitors that were developed to spare mucosal toxicities are used together with L-aspirin, the risk of ulcer hemorrhage has not been shown to increase [1,2,3]. In a recent case-control study by Lanas et al., relative risk of ulcer bleeding during concomitant use of NSAID and L-aspirin was found to be about double that during use of NSAID alone (6.1 vs. 3.3, respectively) [1]. However, no randomized clinical trials have yet compared ulcer incidence between NSAID alone group, concomitant use of NSAID+aspirin and concomitant use of NSAID+NSAID in patients with long-term NSAID administration. Taking our results into consideration, risk of peptic ulcer with concomitant use of L-aspirin does not seem as high as that in RA patients taking NSAID+NSAID.

Effects on Endoscopic Peptic Ulcer by L-Aspirin Co-Therapy With Long-Term Nsaids

From past reports, the prevalence of endoscopic peptic ulcer (defined as an excavated mucosal break ≥3 mm in diameter) is considered to be about 10% in patients taking long-term aspirin and about 20% in patients taking long-term NSAIDs [1,2]. However, no definitive evidence has shown that the presence of endoscopic peptic ulcer is associated with the incidence of ulcer complications. In addition, the point must be made that no prospective long-term studies have shown that treatment targeting endoscopic peptic ulcer can offer efficient prophylaxis of ulcer complication. Goldstein regarded the clinical significance of endoscopic peptic ulcer as questionable [1].

Conversely, as L-aspirin has anti-platelet effect but other NSAIDs do not, L-aspirin-induced endoscopic ulcers may bring about occult hemorrhage even in asymptomatic ulcers without ulcer complication. However, a relationship with occult hemorrhage through endoscopic peptic ulcers and long-term NSAID-aspirin use has not been considered. Most endoscopic peptic ulcers under long-term NSAID treatment are thought to undergo repeated remission and exacerbation. Taking our results into consideration, even if an asymptomatic ulcer is present, L-aspirin with concomitant NSAID use could bring about bleeding. Treatment of endoscopic peptic ulcers under L-aspirin use is expected to contribute to the treatment and prophylaxis of iron-deficiency anemia through potential bleeding. To clarify the clinical significance of endoscopic peptic ulcers in the future, prospective examination is required regarding the associations between endoscopic peptic ulcer and the onset of complication and potential bleeding.

References

[1] Morimoto T, Nakayama M, Saito Y, Ogawa H.Aspirin for primary prevention of atherosclerotic disease in Japan. J Atheroscler Thromb. 2007;14:159-66.

[2] Goldstein JL, Cryer B, Amer F, Hunt B.Celecoxib plus aspirin versus naproxen and lansoprazole plus aspirin: a randomized, double-blind, endoscopic trial. Clin Gastroenterol Hepatol. 2007 ;5:1167-74.

[3] Goldstein JL, Huang B, Amer F, Christopoulos NG.Ulcer recurrence in high-risk patients receiving nonsteroidalanti-inflammatory drugs plus low-dose aspirin: results of a post HOC subanalysis. Clin Ther. 2004;26:1637-43.

[4] Frostegård J: Atherosclerosis in patients with autoimmune disorders. Arterioscler Thromb Vasc Biol 2005, 25:1776-1785.

[5] Solomon DH, Karlson EW, Rimm EB, Cannuscio CC, Mandl LA, Manson JE, Stampfer MJ, Curhan GC: Cardiovascular morbidity and mortality in women diagnosed with rheumatoid arthritis. Circulation 2003, 107:1303-1307.

[6] Wolfe F, Freundlich B, Straus WL: Increase in cardiovascular and cerebrovascular disease prevalence in rheumatoid arthritis. J Rheumatol 2003, 30:36-40.

[7] Del Rincon I, Williams K, Stern MP, Freeman GL, O'Leary DH, Escalante A: Association between carotid atherosclerosis and markers of inflammation in rheumatoid arthritis patients and healthy subjects. Arthritis Rheum 2003, 48:1833-1840.

[8] Dalen JE. Aspirin to prevent heart attack and stroke: what's the right dose? Am J Med. 2006 ;119:198-202.

[9] Weisman SM, Graham DY.Evaluation of the benefits and risks of low-dose aspirin in the secondary prevention of cardiovascular and cerebrovascular events.Arch Intern Med. 2002 ;162:2197-202.

[10] Agrawal NM, Van Kerckhove HE, Erhardt LJ, Geis GS.Misoprostol coadministered with diclofenac for prevention of gastroduodenal ulcers. A one-year study. Dig Dis Sci. 1995;40:1125-31

[11] Roth SH, Tindall EA, Jain AK, McMahon FG, April PA, Bockow BI, Cohen SB, Fleischmann RM.A controlled study comparing the effects of

nabumetone, ibuprofen, and ibuprofen plus misoprostol on the upper gastrointestinal tract mucosa. Arch Intern Med. 1993;153:2565-71.

[12] Taha AS, Hudson N, Hawkey CJ, Swannell AJ, Trye PN, Cottrell J, Mann SG, Simon TJ, Sturrock RD, Russell RI.Famotidine for the prevention of gastric and duodenal ulcers caused by nonsteroidal antiinflammatory drugs. N Engl J Med. 1996;334:1435-9.

[13] Cheatum DE, Arvanitakis C, Gumpel M, Stead H, Geis GS.An endoscopic study of gastroduodenal lesions induced by nonsteroidal anti-inflammatory drugs. Clin Ther. 1999;21:992-1003.

[14] Serrano P, Lanas A, Arroyo MT, Ferreira IJ.Risk of upper gastrointestinal bleeding in patients taking low-dose aspirin for the prevention of cardiovascular diseases. Aliment Pharmacol Ther. 2002;16:1945-53.

[15] Yeomans ND, Lanas AI, Talley NJ, Thomson AB, Daneshjoo R, Eriksson B, Appelman-Eszczuk S, Långström G, Naesdal J, Serrano P, Singh M, Skelly MM, Hawkey CJ. Prevalence and incidence of gastroduodenal ulcers during treatment with vascular protective doses of aspirin. Aliment Pharmacol Ther. 2005 ;22:795-801.

[16] Derry S, Loke YK. Risk of gastrointestinal haemorrhage with long term use of aspirin: meta-analysis.BMJ. 2000;321:1183-7

[17] Sakamoto C, Sugano K, Ota S, Sakaki N, Takahashi S, Yoshida Y, Tsukui T, Osawa H, Sakurai Y, Yoshino J, Mizokami Y, Mine T, Arakawa T, Kuwayama H, Saigenji K, Yakabi K, Chiba T, Shimosegawa T, Sheehan JE, Perez-Gutthann S, Yamaguchi T, Kaufman DW, Sato T, Kubota K, Terano A. Case-control study on the association of upper gastrointestinal bleeding and nonsteroidal anti-inflammatory drugs in Japan. Eur J Clin Pharmacol. 2006;62:765-72.

[18] Taha AS, Angerson WJ, Knill-Jones RP, Blatchford O. Upper gastrointestinal haemorrhage associated with low-dose aspirin and anti-thrombotic drugs - a 6-year analysis and comparison with non-steroidal anti-inflammatory drugs. Aliment Pharmacol Ther. 2005;22:285-9

[19] Fred E. Silverstein, G. Steven Geis, et al Gastrointestinal toxicity with celecoxib vs nonsteroidal anti-inflammatory drugs for osteoarthritis and rheumatoid arthritis : the CLASS study : A randomized controlled trial. Celecoxib Long-term Arthritis Safety Study. : JAMA 2000 ;284:1247-1255

[20] Claire Bombardier, Thomas J. Schnitzer, et al For the VIGOR Study Group : Comparison of upper gastrointestinal toxicity of rofecoxib and

naproxen in patients with rheumatoid arthritis. VIGOR Study Group. : N Eugl J Med 2000 ;343:1520-1528

[21] Rick A. Weideman, Kevin C. Kelly, Salahuddin Kazi, Anh Cung, Kevin W. Roberts, Herbert J. Smith, George A. Sarosi, Jr, Bertis B. Little, Byron Cryer. Risks of clinically significant upper gastrointestinal events with etodolac and naproxen: A historical cohort analysis. Gastroenterology. 2004 ;127:1322-1328

[22] Garcia Rodriguez LA, Barreales Tolosa L. Risk of upper gastrointestinal complications among users of traditional NSAIDs and COXIBs in the general population. Gastroenterology. 2007 ;132:498-506

[23] Goldstein JL, Lowry SC, Lanza FL, Schwartz HI, Dodge WE. The impact of low-dose aspirin on endoscopic gastric and duodenal ulcer rates in users of a non-selective non-steroidal anti-inflammatory drug or a cyclo-oxygenase-2-selective inhibitor. Aliment Pharmacol Ther. 2006;23:1489-98.

[24] Sørensen HT, Mellemkjaer L, Blot WJ, Nielsen GL, Steffensen FH, McLaughlin JK, Olsen JH. Risk of upper gastrointestinal bleeding associated with use of low-dose aspirin. Am J Gastroenterol. 2000;95:2218-24.

[25] Lanas A, García-Rodríguez LA, Arroyo MT, Gomollón F, Feu F, González-Pérez A, Zapata E, Bástida G, Rodrigo L, Santolaria S, Güell M, de Argila CM, Quintero E, Borda F, Piqué JM; Asociación Española de Gastroenterología.Risk of upper gastrointestinal ulcer bleeding associated with selective cyclo-oxygenase-2 inhibitors, traditional non-aspirin non-steroidal anti-inflammatory drugs, aspirin and combinations. Gut. 2006;55:1731-8.

[26] Cheatum DE, Arvanitakis C, Gumpel M, Stead H, Geis GS.An endoscopic study of gastroduodenal lesions induced by nonsteroidal anti-inflammatory drugs.Clin Ther. 1999;21:992-1003.

[27] Yeomans ND, Lanas AI, Talley NJ, Thomson AB, Daneshjoo R, Eriksson B, Appelman-Eszczuk S, Långström G, Naesdal J, Serrano P, Singh M, Skelly MM, Hawkey CJ.Prevalence and incidence of gastroduodenal ulcers during treatment with vascular protective doses of aspirin. Aliment Pharmacol Ther. 2005 ;22:795-801.

[28] [1] Goldstein JL.Who needs prophylaxis of nonsteroidal anti-inflammatory drug-induced ulcers and what is optimal prophylaxis?Eur J Gastroenterol Hepatol. 2000 ;12:S11-5.

In: Ulcers: Causes, Diagnosis, and Treatment ISBN: 978-1-60741-253-3
Editors: Danijel Erceg et al. pp. 37-41

Chapter 3

NEW HORIZON IN THE TREATMENT OF PERFORATED PEPTIC ULCER

Isidoro Di Carlo*[*]*, Elia Pulvirenti and Adriana Toro
Department of Surgical Sciences, Organ Transplantation and Advanced Technologies, University of Catania, Cannizzaro Hospital, Catania, Italy

Gastric or duodenal perforation is a serious complication of peptic ulcer, with a poor prognosis especially in the elderly [1].

Data shows women affected the most, perhaps because of an increased consumption of non-steroidal anti-inflammatory drugs [2]. Diabetes and cardiovascular or pulmonary diseases can increase the mortality if associated with the preoperative shock and a perforation time longer than 48h [3].

Surgery for peptic ulcer perforation is one of the most common emergency procedures carried out in the Western world [4] and, over the past decades, many technical modifications to standard perforated peptic ulcer (PPU) repair have been described to make the operation safer and to reduce morbidity and mortality rates. However, its mortality risk remains significantly high, despite improvement in surgical techniques, anesthesia and critical care, a better understanding of the pathophysiology of the disease, and the wide availability of antibiotics [5]. This risk is assessed to be around 30% [6], rising

* Corresponding Author: Department of Surgical Sciences, Organ Transplantation, and Advanced Technologies, University of Catania, Cannizzaro Hospital, Via Messina, 95126 Catania, Italy. Tel.: +39 095 7264863. Fax: +39 095 7263020. E-mail: idicarlo@unict.it

to almost 100% in elderly patients with coexisting illnesses who experience more than a 24h delay before surgical treatment [7]. Indeed, the early diagnoses and early treatment are two basic factors influencing the prognosis of patients with PPU, especially the elderly [1]: the risk of death for sepsis is very high in patients who had undergone emergency surgery after a long waiting period (because of the absence of intestinal preparation and the exposure of the peritoneal serosa to the gastric acid for a long time [1].

When gastric perforation occurs, abdominal x-ray examination shows free intraperitoneal air between the diaphragm and liver, but if much time passes, almost all this air is absorbed, so a CT-scan is necessary to diagnose the perforation [8].

The first successful surgical management of PPU disease was described during the late 19th century, but which is the best surgical procedure is still debatable. Options range from damage control without addressing the main pathology to the definitive management of PPU disease [5]. Today, the gold standard for treatment of such perforations is the pedicle omental patch, first described by Celan-Jones in 1929, although it is commonly attributed to Graham, who described the use of a free graft of the omentum to repair the perforation in 1937. In this, a strand of omentum is drawn over the perforation and held in place by full thickness sutures placed on either side of the perforation [9].

With this approach, mortality is significantly associated with the following factors: age, time delay between perforation and operation, presence of comorbid conditions, respiratory and pulse rate, raised blood urea and serum creatinine, size of perforation, amount of peritoneal fluid, and requirement of postoperative intensive care unit support [10-11].

Occasionally, especially in the presence of large perforations, other surgical options may be necessary for adequate closure and to avoid fistulas formation: partial gastrectomy, jejunal serosal patch or pedicle graft, free omental plug, proximal gastrojejunostomy or gastric disconnection [9].

Also, laparoscopic perforation closure can be performed effectively with Graham's patch omentoplasty, as in conventional surgery; with the advent of minimal access techniques, laparoscopy has been used for the treatment of this condition since 1990 [12]. Laparoscopic repair is associated with lesser postoperative analgesic use, decreased hospital stay (the postoperative hospitalization period using the open technique is approximately 13 days [13]), lower wound infection, and decreased mortality rate.

Since the initial reports of successful laparoscopic management of PPU disease, several comparative series have been published confirming the technical feasibility and demonstrating some of the advantages of this approach [14]. Despite the appeal of the minimally invasive surgery, no definitive criteria have been established to select patients who may benefit the most from this approach and those in whom its use is contraindicated, especially today, with the effectiveness of the antiulcer medications [14]

Moreover, a nonjuxtapyloric gastric ulcer, an ulcer greater than 10mm in diameter, delayed surgery for more than 24h, major medical illnesses, shock at admission, and patients with technical difficulties should be avoided with the laparoscopic approach [15]. On the other hand, open repair is associated with reduced operating time and a lower reoperation rate after repair [16].

Over the past decades, many technical changes to the traditional Graham technique have been described in the literature, but there is no reference to the use of a fibrinogen- and thrombin-coated collagen patch for a PPU. The patch is a device originally intended to be employed in hepatic resections and kidney surgery [17] to make rapid and lasting hemostasis, but it is also used after thoracic surgery to avoid air leak after lung resections [18]. It is constituted by a matrix of equine collagen coated with human fibrinogen and thrombin. It does not contain bovine components, avoiding the risk of transmission of prion disease such as Creutzfeldt-Jakob disease. It is also treated to inactivate viruses such as HIV, HAV, HBV, and HCV. The sponge works by simulating the last step of the coagulation cascade: the thrombin converts the fibrinogen into fibrin monomers, whose polymerization and stabilization generate a hemostatic coating. Coagulation occurs both inside the collagen matrix and on the tissue interruption. The effective hemostasis is activated in 3-5min and the sponge is degraded in 12 weeks through fibrinolysis and phagocytosis [19].

During hepatic surgery, this device shows a strong tightness, especially in the early postoperative period, when the sponge generated fluid collection underneath its layer, without liquid leakage or hemorrhage. This observation induced to extend its use also for gastric perforation in association with Graham's traditional technique.

The surgical technique to apply the patch is the following: under general anesthesia, the access to the abdominal wall is obtained through a xifo-umbilical incision; after the individuation of the perforation, the gastric wall is repaired by a full thickness suture, followed by collagen patch application, which is finally covered by the classic omental patch.

The sponge should be applied by covering 1–2cm over the interruption of the gastric wall and the device results are completely effective only after a pressure of 3–5min.

In laparoscopy, this approach provides the suture of the gastric wall followed only by a sponge application and avoiding the omental patch preparation and its suture. To be effective, also in laparoscopy the device must be maintained pressured for 3–5min with a paddle retractor.

The fibrinogen- and thrombin-coated collagen patch may improve the seal of the traditional repair, has no complications, and makes the overall operation faster, resulting in time-sparing treatment especially in laparoscopy. However, further studies and follow-up are needed before considering extensive use of this technical modification.

REFERENCES

[29] Di Carlo, I; Toro, A; Sparatore, F; Primo, S; Barbagallo, F; Di Blasi, M. Emergency gastric ulcer complications in elderly. Factors affecting the morbidity and mortality in relation to therapeutic approaches. *Minerva Chir*. 2006, 61, 325-32.

[30] Fowler, SF; Khoubian, JF; Mathiasen, RA; Margulies, DR. Peptic ulcers in the elderly is a surgical disease. *Am J Surg*., 2001, 182, 733-7.

[31] Scott Jones, R. Acute abdomen. In: Sabiston DC, Jr., editor. *Textbook of Surgery: The biological basis of modern surgical practice*. Philadelphia: *WB Saunders Company*, 2001, 48, 156-62.

[32] Sweeney, KJ; Faolain, MO; Gannon, D; Gorey, TF; Kerin, MJ. Surgical management of perforated peptic ulcer disease. *Ir J Med Sci,* 2006, 175, 50-54.

[33] Rahman, MM; Islam, MS; Flora, S; Akhter, SF; Hossain, S; Karim, F; Mortality in perforated peptic ulcer patients after selective management of stratified poor risk cases. *World J Surg,* 2007, 31, 2341-2344.

[34] Barut, I; Tarhan, OR; Cerci, C; Karaguzel, N; Akdeniz, Y; Bulbul, M. Prognostic factors of peptic ulcer perforation. *Saudi Med J,* 2005, 26, 1255-1259.

[35] Taha, AS; Angerson, WJ; Prasad, R; McCloskey, C; Gilmour, D; Morran, CG. The incidence and early mortality after peptic ulcer perforation and the use of low-dose aspirin and non-steroidal anti-inflammatory drugs. *Aliment Pharmacol Ther,* 2008, 1, 28, 878-85.

[36] Tsugawa, K; Koyanagi, N; Hashizume, M; Tomikawa, M; Akahoshi, K; Ayukawa, K; Wada, H; Tanoue, K; Sugimachi, K. The therapeutic strategies in performing emergency surgery for gastroduodenal ulcer

perforation in 130 patients over 70 years of age. *Hepatogastroenterology.*, 2001, 48, 156-62.

[37] Gupta, S; Kaushik, R; Sharma, R; Attri, A. The management of large perforations of duodenal ulcers. *BMC Surg,* 2005, 5, 15.

[38] Subedi, SK; Afaq, A; Adhikary, S; Niraula, SR; Agrawal, CS. Factors influencing mortality in perforated duodenal ulcer following emergency surgical repair. *JNMA J Nepal Med Assoc,* 2007, 46, 31-35.

[39] Arici, C; Mesci, A; Dincer, D; Dinckan, A; Colak, T. Analysis of risk factors predicting (affecting) mortality and morbidity of peptic ulcer perforations. *Int Surg,* 2007, 92, 147-154.

[40] Nathanson, LK; Easter, DW; Cuschieri, A. Laparoscopic repair/peritoneal toilet of perforated duodenal ulcer. *Surg Endosc,* 1990, 4, 232-233.

[41] Bin-Taleb, AK; Razzaq, RA; Al-Kathiri, ZO. Management of perforated peptic ulcer in patients at a teaching hospital. *Saudi Med J,* 2008, 29, 245-250.

[42] Katkhouda, N; Mavor, E; Mason, RJ; Campos, GM; Soroushyari, A; Berne, TV. Laparoscopic repair of perforated duodenal ulcers: outcome and efficacy in 30 consecutive patients. *Arch Surg.*, 1999, 134, 845-8,

[43] Ates, M; Sevil, S; Bakircioglu, E; Colak, C. Laparoscopic repair of peptic ulcer perforation without omental patch versus conventional open repair. *J Laparoendosc Adv Surg Tech A,* 2007, 17, 615-619.

[44] Palanivelu, C; Jani, K; Senthilnathan, P. Laparoscopic management of duodenal ulcer perforation: is it advantageous? *Indian J Gastroenterol,* 2007, 26, 64-66.

[45] Attar, KH; Namasivayam, J; Green, J; Peters, J. Kidney salvage using the fibrinogen- and thrombin-coated sponge TachoSil during nephron-sparing surgery for the resection of large renal tumours. *Ann R Coll Surg Engl,* 2008, 90, W8-W11.

[46] Anegg, U; Lindenmann, J; Matzi, V; Smolle, J; Maier, A; Smolle-Jüttner, F. Efficiency of fleece-bound sealing (TachoSil) of air leaks in lung surgery: a prospective randomised trial. *Eur J Cardiothorac Surg,* 2007, 31, 198-202.

[47] Frilling, A; Stavrou, GA; Mischinger, HJ; de Hemptinne, B; Rokkjaer, M; Klempnauer, J; Thörne, A; Gloor, B; Beckebaum, S; Ghaffar, MF; Broelsch, CE. Effectiveness of a new carrier-bound fibrin sealant versus argon beamer as haemostatic agent during liver resection: a randomised prospective trial. *Langenbecks Arch Surg,* 2005, 390, 114-120.

In: Ulcers: Causes, Diagnosis, and Treatment ISBN: 978-1-60741-253-3
Editors: Danijel Erceg et al. pp. 43-63

Chapter 4

EFFECT OF GENDER AND SMOKING ON INCIDENCE OF CARDIOVASCULAR DISEASE AND PEPTIC ULCER IN A JAPANESE POPULATION: THE RADIATION EFFECTS RESEARCH FOUNDATION ADULT HEALTH STUDY

Michiko Yamada[1] and F. Lennie Wong[2]

Departments of [1]Clinical Studies and [2]Statistics,
Radiation Effects Research Foundation, Japan

ABSTRACT

Background

Studies on the effects of gender and smoking on cardiovascular and peptic ulcer disease have been reported in Western countries, but data from Asian countries are limited and inconsistent.

Methods

We examined the effects of gender and smoking on cardiovascular and peptic ulcer disease using the longitudinal data of the Adult Health Study collected during biennial health examinations from 1 July 1958 to 30 June 1998. The examinations included medical history, chest x-ray, ultrasonography, and fluoroscopy or endoscopy. Smoking histories were obtained from 5 questionnaires self-administered during different time periods. We estimated the relative risks for being female and for "ever" versus "never" smoking after adjusting for significant effects of age, city, birth cohort, calendar time, alcohol intake, and radiation dose. We also examined the interaction between gender and smoking.

Results

Eight hundred and fifty four strokes, 215 aortic aneurysms, 1093 gastric ulcers, and 437 duodenal ulcers were detected between 1958 to 1998: and, from 1978 to 1998, 125 myocardial infarction were detected. The incidence of myocardial infarction, stroke, and gastric and duodenal ulcer was significantly higher in men than in women, but we found no gender difference for aortic aneurysm incidence after adjustment for smoking status. We detected positive associations of smoking with myocardial infarction (RR for ever smoked to never smoked, 1.96), stroke (RR, 1.26), aortic aneurysm (RR, 1.80), gastric ulcer (RR, 2.06), and duodenal ulcer (RR, 1.32). The interaction between gender and smoking status was not significant for any of the diseases.

Conclusions

Male gender and smoking were significant risk factors for cardiovascular and peptic ulcer disease in a Japanese population.

Keywords: Gender differences, smoking, myocardial infarction, stroke, aortic aneurysm, gastric ulcer, duodenal ulcer

INTRODUCTION

Many epidemiological studies in Western populations have reported gender differences for, and smoking effects on, cardiovascular disease and peptic ulcers.[1-5] Studies regarding stroke and coronary heart disease from

Asian populations are limited, however, and the results are inconsistent.[6-10] Incidence and risk factor studies on peptic ulcers and aortic aneurysm in Asia are also limited.

Previous investigations on the relationship between cardiovascular disease and smoking in Japan varied by design (cross-sectional, case-control, and prospective studies), study population (gender, age, general population, and outpatient), or endpoint (mortality and incidence). The 23-year follow-up of the Hisayama study (a long-term prospective study of rural Japanese subjects followed since 1961) showed that cigarette smoking was an independent and significant risk factor for coronary heart disease, but not for non-embolic cerebral infarction.[6] Other pre-1980 Japanese epidemiological studies found no association between smoking and stroke.[7, 11, 12] The 32-year follow-up of the Hisayama study reported that smoking was a risk factor for lacunar stroke, the most common type of cerebral infarction in their study.[8] Studies published after the 1980s showed that smoking raised the risk of stroke [9, 13] and myocardial infarction (MI).[14] Only the Hisayama study reported gender differences in the incidence of all types of cardiovascular disease[6] and the prevalence of coronary atherosclerosis in the Japanese population.[15]

The Honolulu heart program, a long-term prospective study that has been following Japanese-American men in Hawaii since 1965, provided evidence that smoking was a risk factor for stroke, coronary heart disease, aortic aneurysm, and peptic ulcer.[16-19]

Although many studies report gender-specific estimates of incidence and mortality rates and gender-specific smoking effects on cardiovascular disease and peptic ulcer, gender differences have not been examined formally. In this study, we examined the effects of gender and smoking on the incidence of MI, stroke, aortic aneurysm, gastric ulcer, and duodenal ulcer in the Radiation Effects Research Foundation (RERF) Adult Health Study (AHS) cohort. The AHS has health data spanning from 1958 to1998 for one of the largest existing cohorts of middle-aged and elderly men and women,[20, 21] and it is still ongoing.

Subjects and Methods

Subjects

The AHS was begun in 1958 by the Atomic Bomb Casualty Commission and was succeeded in 1975 by the Radiation Effects Research Foundation (RERF). By providing biennial clinical examinations to atomic-bomb survivors and their controls in Hiroshima and Nagasaki, the AHS has tracked the long-term clinical effects of exposure to atomic-bomb radiation.[20, 21]

Table 1. Characteristics of study subjects

		Hiroshima		Nagasaki	
		Men	Women	Men	Women
Total		2984	5265	1561	2172
Age in 1945	Mean	31.0	30.0	25.5	23.6
S.D.		15.9	14.6	14.7	13.0
Age at examination	Range	13 – 92	13 – 98	14 – 98	14 – 97
Smoking	Never smoked	300 (10%)	3709 (70%)	205 (13%)	1658 (76%)
	Ever smoked	2366 (79%)	996 (19%)	1258 (80%)	364 (17%)
	Missing data	318 (11%)	560 (11%)	98 (6%)	150 (7%)
Drinking	Never drank	472 (16%)	3180 (60%)	272 (17%)	1530 (70%)
	Ever drank	2076 (70%)	1440 (27%)	1132 (73%)	464 (21%)
	Missing data	436 (15%)	645 (12%)	157 (10%)	178 (8%)
Number of cases	Total				
Myocardial infarction[a]	125	50	40	17	18
Stroke	854	291	312	142	109
Aortic aneurysm	215	60	88	31	36
Gastric ulcer	1093	394	394	182	123
Duodenal ulcer	438	169	115	94	59
Radiation dose	Dose=0	1003 (34%)	1746 (33%)	514 (33%)	691(32%)
	Mean (Sv)	0.38	0.33	0.41	0.40
	Missing	286 (10%)	388 (7%)	450 (29%)	519 (24%)

a for incidence during 1978-1998.
Parenthetical values represent %.

The subjects of the present analysis are the 11,982 who attended at least two AHS examinations between 1 July 1958 and 30 June 1998 (about half of the original AHS subjects had died by then). About 62% of the participants were women and 69% were Hiroshima residents (Table 1). A high participation rate (75% to 90%) has been maintained, and more than half of the study participants underwent 11 or more routine clinical examinations.

Clinical Procedures and Selection of Diseases for Study

All participants provided informed consent, and the study complied with institutional guidelines regarding research ethics and the welfare of human subjects. A detailed description of the clinical procedures is available elsewhere.[20, 21] Briefly, the biennial AHS examination includes a clinical history taking, a physical examination, blood pressure measurements, urinalysis, blood cell count, biochemical tests, a chest X-ray, an electrocardiogram, and ultrasonography. Diagnoses were encoded according to the International Classification of Diseases (ICD)[22] and entered into the AHS database. The first 3 digits of the ICD codes (up to 6 diagnoses per person) were stored until June 1986, and 4-digit codes (up to 12 per person) were stored thereafter (appendix). MI was determined by history of hospitalization or angiography with a diagnosis of MI, episode of chest pain, and development of ischemic change on electrocardiogram. Stroke was determined by history of hospitalization or CT/MRI examination with a diagnosis of stroke and episode of neurological deficit. MI was not ascertained prior to July 1978 because ICD codes for acute MI and old MI did not exist then. Aortic aneurysm (thoracic and abdominal aortic aneurysm and aortic dissection) was diagnosed by medical history, chest x-ray examination, and ultrasonography. Ultrasonography was used optionally from 1981 to 1990 in Hiroshima and from 1984 to 1990 in Nagasaki. Since 1991, it has been performed routinely. It should be noted that this study includes only survivors of MI, stroke, ruptured aortic aneurysm, and aortic dissection who underwent subsequent examinations, as death certificate data were not considered. About 5% of participants, however, underwent clinical examinations at home or in a nearby hospital or an institution where they were residing because of severe illness or advanced age. Peptic ulcer was diagnosed by medical history and fluoroscopy or endoscopy, which were conducted optionally for subjects whose stool occult blood test was positive in a routine examination.

Cigarette Smoking and Alcohol Consumption Data

We obtained cigarette smoking history from 5 questionnaires self-administered to men in 1965, to women in 1969-1970, and to both men and women in 1965-1966, 1979-1980, and 1991. The response rate was over 95% for all surveys. Due to differences in the questionnaires and the make-up of the survey participants, the subjects were classified simply as "never smoked" (i.e., indicated in all the surveys that they had never smoked), "ever smoked" (indicated in any survey that they had smoked some quantity of cigarettes), or "missing smoking data" (did not participate in any of the smoking surveys).

Alcohol intake information was obtained from 3 questionnaires self-administered to both sexes in 1965-1966, 1979-1980, and 1991. The same classifications were applied: never drank, ever drank, and missing data. Non-drinkers were subjects who did not drink any beer, whiskey, shochu (Japanese distilled liquor), wine (including sake), or other liquor.

Statistical Methods

We applied Poisson regression methods for the longitudinal analysis of incidence data using AMFIT from the EPICURE program package.[23] We based person-year calculations on the subject's follow-up period, which began at the initial AHS visit and ended on the last disease-free visit or the date of disease onset, whichever came earlier. We estimated the disease onset date as the midpoint between the date of the initial AHS exam with a positive diagnosis and the date of the previous disease-free examination. For each disease, we excluded prevalent cases at the initial visit. We cross-tabulated person-years and case counts by stratifying the following covariates: city (Hiroshima, Nagasaki), sex (male, female), age at examination in years (0–39, 40–49, 50–59, 60–69, 70+), age at the time of the atomic bombings in years (0–9, 10–19, 20–29, 30–39, 40+), calendar time (1 July 1958 to 30 June 1978, 1 July 1978 to 30 June 1998), cigarette smoking (never smoked, ever smoked, missing data), alcohol consumption status (never drank, ever drank, missing data), and atomic-bomb radiation dose using the DS86 weighted stomach dose in Sv (missing, 0, 0.001–0.49, 0.5–1.49, 1.50+). Significant dose effects were not demonstrated in the previous AHS report for the diseases considered here.[20, 21] A detailed description of the dose estimation is available elsewhere.[21]

We modeled the disease incidence rates (γ) parametrically using the exponential function, $\gamma(x_1, \ldots, x_c) = \exp\{\sum_i \beta_i x_i\}$, where x_i is a covariable. We treated covariates as categorical except for age at the time of the bombings and age at examination, for which we used the cell-specific means. We included up to the third power of mean age at examination and at the time of the bombings in order to adjust for potential non-linear age effects. We allowed only the significant covariates in the model and considered first order interactions. We computed the relative risks (RRs) of a covariate using models that did not include its interactions with age at time of the bombings or age at examination. We calculated the RR based on indicator variables for the covariates in the models. We used the likelihood ratio method to test the significance of the coefficients of the covariates using Type I error rate of .05, in a forward step-wise algorithm, and to compute the 95% confidence intervals.

RESULTS

Table 1 shows the characteristics of study subjects by gender and city. Overall among men, 11% never smoked, 80% ever smoked, and smoking data were missing for 9%; 16% never drank, 70% ever drank, and drinking data were missing for 13%. Overall among women, 72% never smoked, 18% ever smoked, and smoking data were missing for 10%; 63% never drank, 26% ever drank, and drinking data were missing for 11%. The distribution of smokers by atomic bomb radiation exposure did not vary significantly for men ($P = 0.14$), but there were significantly more smokers among the exposed women than among the non-exposed women (23% vs. 17%; $P < 0.0001$). The distribution of drinkers did not vary significantly by radiation exposure for either sex (data not shown).

Table 2 shows the number of incident cases and crude incidence rates for MI, stroke, aortic aneurysm, gastric ulcer, and duodenal ulcer by each variable and the multivariate adjusted RRs. Crude incidence rates were higher for men for all diseases, and RRs were significantly lower for women for all diseases, except aortic aneurysm. Risk for aortic aneurysm was same in males and females. Although the incidence of aortic aneurysm was significantly lower for women when smoking was not included in the model ($P = 0.008$), the gender difference was not significant when smoking status was included ($P = 0.42$).

We detected a significantly increased RR for ever smokers compared with never smokers for all diseases, while the interaction between gender and smoking status was not significant for any of diseases (p-values=0.29, 0.81, 0.41, 0.16, and 0.44, respectively for MI, stroke, aortic aneurysm, gastric ulcer, and duodenal ulcer). Hiroshima residents showed a higher incidence of gastric ulcer. The younger birth cohort showed a higher incidence of gastric ulcer and duodenal ulcer. A higher incidence among older subjects was found for all diseases except duodenal ulcer, which displayed a convex risk curve (Figure 1).

Table 2. Multivariate adjusted relative risks for myocardial infarction, stroke, aortic aneurysm, gastric ulcer, and duodenal ulcer

Disease	Myocardial infarction[a]	Stroke	Aortic aneurysm	Gastric ulcer	Duodenal ulcer
Number of cases	125	854	215	1093	437
Males	67	433	91	576	263
Females	58	421	124	517	174
Person-years	111930	289629	293634	279650	287700
Males	36382	100183	102330	94738	98279
Female	75548	189446	191304	184912	189421
Crude incidence rate (10,000 PY)	11.2	29.5	7.3	39.1	15.2
Males	18.4	43.2	8.9	60.8	26.8
Females	7.7	22.2	6.5	28.0	9.2
Relative risk					
Sex (Female to Male, age 50)	0.59	0.54	0.99	0.71	0.43
(95% confidence interval)	(0.37 – 0.94)	(0.46 – 0.64)	(0.70 – 1.39)	(0.61 – 0.83)	(0.33 – 0.56)
P-value	0.025	<0.001	0.97	<0.001	<0.001
Smoking (Ever to Never)	1.96	1.26	1.80	2.06	1.32
(95% confidence interval)	(1.20 – 3.16)	(1.05 - 1.51)	(1.37 – 2.37)	(1.75 - 2.42)	(1.01 - 1.72)
P-value	0.018	0.013	<0..001	<0.001	0.043
City (Nagasaki to Hiroshima)	0.75	1.04	1.14	0.76	0.95
P-value	0.14	0.62	0.38	<0.0001	0.62
Period (late to early[b])	-	1.11	0.92	0.92	0.95

P-value	-	0.15	0.57	0.60	0.84
Drinking (Ever to Never)	0.83	0.93	0.90	1.01	1.06
P-value	0.39	0.36	0.50	0.38	0.50
Age in 1945					
15	1.00	1.00	1.00	1.00	1.00
25	0.74	0.95	1.06	0.90	0.86
35	0.54	0.90	1.13	0.81	0.74
45	0.40	0.86	1.20	0.73	0.63
Disease	Myocardial infarction[a]	Stroke	Aortic aneurysm	Gastric ulcer	Duodenal ulcer
P-value	0.17	0.16	0.42	0.003	0.010
Age at examination					
45	1.00	1.00	1.00	1.00	1.00
55	1.76	3.71	2.91	1.19	0.91
65	3.10	10.57	8.51	1.25	0.66
75	5.46	18.21	16.88	1.17	0.39
P-value	<0.0001	<0.0001	<0.0001	<0.0001	<0.0001

a Incidence, 1978-1998; b Early period, 7/58 – 6/78; late period, 7/78 – 6/98.

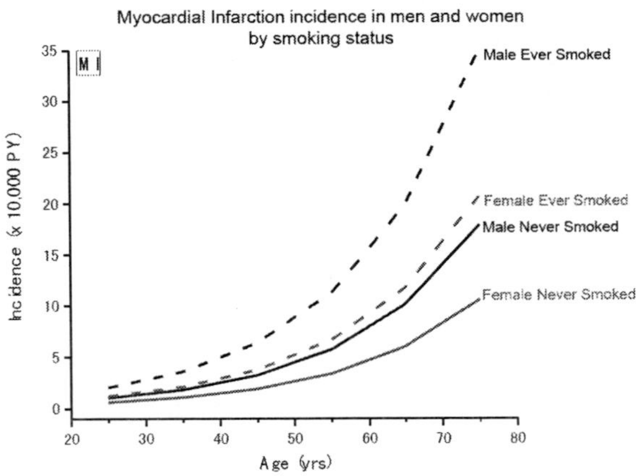

Figure 1. (*Continued*)

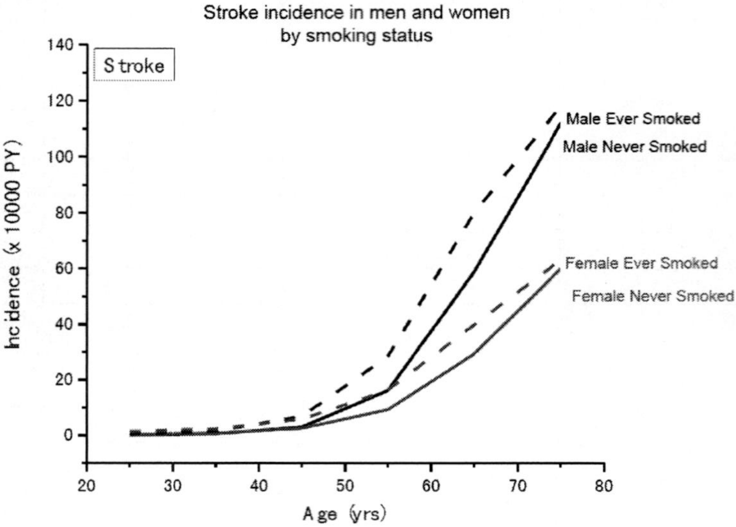

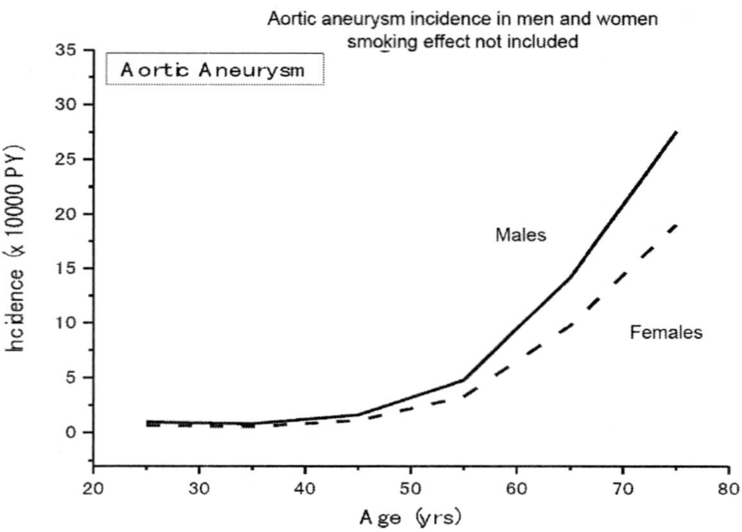

Figure 1. (*Continued*)

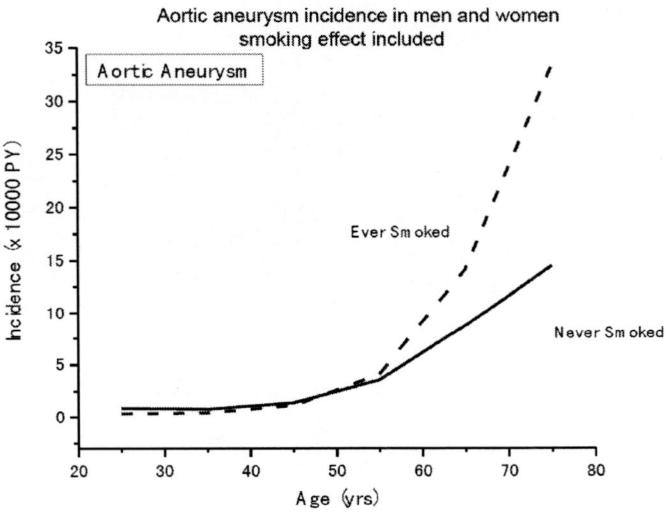

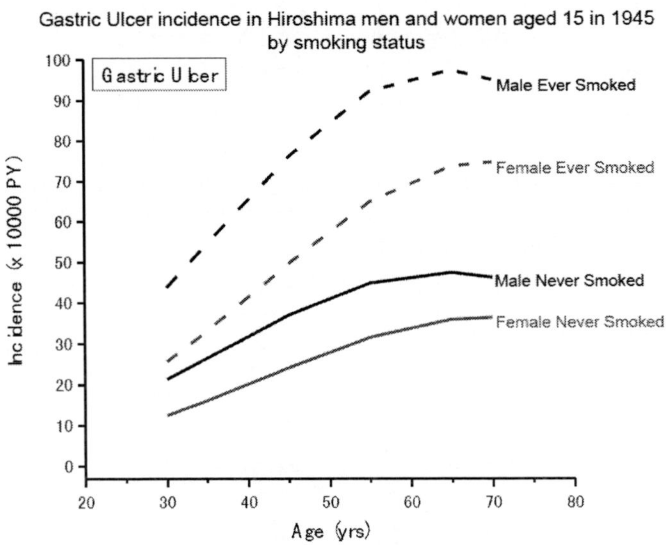

Figure 1. (*Continued*)

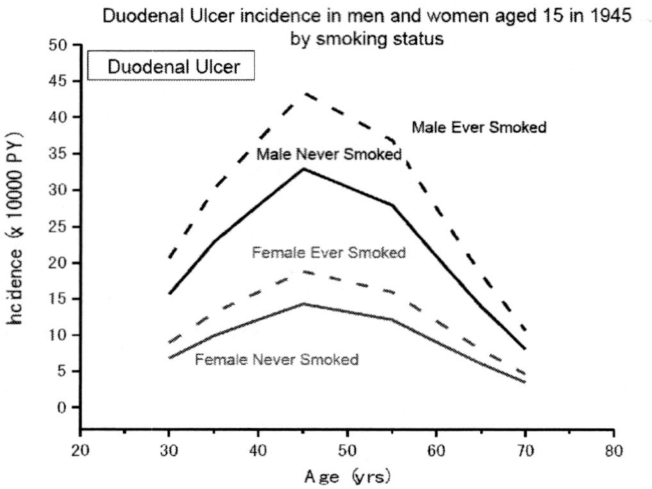

Figure 1. Gender-age specific incidence for myocardial infarction, stroke, aortic aneurysm, gastric ulcer, and duodenal ulcer.

Figure 1 shows the fitted age-specific incidence curves for MI, stroke, and gastric and duodenal ulcer by gender and smoking status. Because gender difference was significant for aortic aneurysm before, but not after adjustment for smoking status, age-specific incidence for aortic aneurysm by gender is shown unadjusted for smoking. The incidence curves by smoking status are also shown. The effects were significant, independent of gender. Adjusted for the significant covariates for each disease, we plotted the incidence of MI and duodenal ulcer in both cities, and of gastric ulcer for Hiroshima, for men and women aged 15 in 1945. Incidence of MI, stroke, aortic aneurysm, and gastric ulcer increased significantly with age. Incidence of duodenal ulcer peaked in the 4th and 5th decades of life and then declined. Incidence of duodenal ulcer peaked later in older cohorts.

DISCUSSION

In this prospective study of a large Japanese cohort, the crude incidence rates for MI, stroke, and aortic aneurysm were higher for men than for women, but the RR was higher only for MI and stroke after adjustment for smoking status. Similar RRs for stroke were reported previously in Japan [6, 24] and Europe, [25, 26] and a smaller RR was reported in the US.[27] Although the gender difference in MI morbidity tended to diminish after menopausal age in the Framingham study, [28] we found no such tendency. A limitation in our study, however, was that some cases of silent MI, and all cases of fatal MI and stroke, were not included because some medical charts were not validated and death certificate data were not considered. The MI incidence in the AHS in 1958 and 1984 was calculated using a stringent set of criteria, including a review of medical history, electrocardiogram results, death certificate data, and autopsy information, was 1.6 times higher in men than in women.[29] In another AHS study that used similar criteria, the incidence of stroke and coronary heart disease, including asymptomatic and fatal cases, was twice as high in men as in women.[30] The risk of abdominal aortic aneurysm was about two times higher for men than for women in the Chicago Heart Association cohort.[31] The mortality rate of aortic aneurysm in Japan and its incidence rate (based on ultrasound scanning) in Malaysia were also more than twice as high in men.[32, 33] To clarify the disparity in the gender effect on aortic aneurysm that depended on smoking adjustment in this study, we examined the gender-specific crude incidence rates in the never smoked and the ever smoked groups. Whereas the crude incidence rate was higher for male never smokers than for female never smokers (7.97 vs. 5.32 per 10,000 py), it was lower for male ever smokers than for female ever smokers (8.96 vs. 11.36). A plausible explanation for our not detecting a gender difference in aortic aneurysm incidence after adjustment for smoking is that the proportion of fatal cases might have been higher among male smokers than among female smokers. The explanation is supported by the observation that male smokers have an increased risk of aneurysm rupture and poorer long-term survival.[34, 35] A future analysis that includes fatal cases should serve to clarify gender differences in cardiovascular disease within this cohort.

We found the incidence of peptic ulcer to be higher among men than among women, which is consistent with previous studies of Japanese and Koreans in Japan.[36, 37] Although more pronounced risks were seen in men in Western societies before the 1970s, [38] recent studies in Europe and in the US show a more equal distribution of peptic ulcer incidence between the sexes.[39, 40]

The smoking information we used in this study was obtained from multiple questionnaires administered over some time and could reflect changing habits. The lack of detailed temporal information necessitated our lumping current and past smokers into an "ever smoked" category. However, it is possible that the never smoked group may have contained a few subjects who started smoking after the last questionnaire was administered and that the ever smoked group included subjects who quit smoking over 5 years previously. Moreover, since the number of cigarettes smoked was not available in this study, we could not perform dose-response analyses.

The disease incidences for the ever smoked in this study were significantly higher than that for the never smoked, although the RR estimates (Table 2) were lower than those for current smoker versus nonsmoker reported in other studies.[3, 13, 14, 18, 19, 36, 41] Since smoking cessation and fewer smoking years are important for reducing the risk of cardiovascular disease and peptic ulcer,[4, 42-46] the lower RRs seen in this study may be due to the ever smoked category containing some current smokers.

Case ascertainment in this study was limited to participants whose illness was not fatal or too severe to preclude study participation. This may have led to an underestimation of smoker risk since illnesses in smokers tend to be of greater severity.[15, 47, 48] Although we did not consider in this analysis hypertension and diabetes, both well-known risk factors for cardiovascular disease, higher blood pressure among smokers has been observed in our cohort,[49] and smoking is associated with an increased risk of type 2 diabetes among middle-aged and elderly Japanese men and women.[50] Thus the smoking effects estimated in this study included both direct effects and indirect effects of confounding risk factors. Despite those limitations, we believe that our data clearly show that smoking negatively impacts the health of the cohort through the onset of these diseases.

Lederle's systematic review [51] of studies that examined smoking effects on aortic aneurysm and other smoking-related diseases showed that association of aortic aneurysm with smoking was greater than for MI or stroke. The RR estimate for aortic aneurysm in the present study was much lower than in previous studies based on both mortality and incidence. Further, there was no pronounced effect of smoking on aortic aneurysm.

The RR for individuals in the ever smoked category, relative to the never smoked category was higher for gastric ulcer than for duodenal ulcer, which is consistent with findings from other studies of Japanese [36, 37] and Japanese-Americans in Hawaii.[19] On the other hand, the RR was slightly greater for duodenal ulcer than for gastric ulcer among European countries.[52, 53] Our finding that the crude incidence rate was higher for gastric ulcer than for duodenal ulcer was consistent with reports from other Japanese populations [36, 37] and Japanese-Americans,[19] but not those from European countries.[53, 54] The US National Health Interview Survey [40] reported that duodenal ulcer was more common in whites than non-whites, while gastric ulcer was more common in non-whites. *Helicobacter pylori* infection, a major risk for peptic ulcer, [53] may be an important factor for interpreting apparent racial differences, since the prevalence of *H. pylori* infection is much higher in Japan and Asia than in Europe.[55] In Japan, the prevalence of *H. pylori* infection was high for those born before 1950 and decreased in later birth cohorts as Japan became more Westernized.[56, 57] Our study participants were all born in, or before 1945,. In this cohort, the prevalence of a positive IgG antibody response to *H. pylori* was about 60% in 2000 and 2002.[58] Since early acquisition of *H. pylori* increases the risk for developing gastric but not duodenal ulcer,[59] the higher prevalence of early *H. pylori* infection in Japan might have led to an increase in gastric ulcer incidence. Further analysis is required to fully elucidate the difference in incidence patterns and smoking effects on gastric and duodenal ulcer.

Although we found a greater incidence rate for MI, stroke, and peptic ulcer in men, the effects of smoking were comparable in both sexes. The incidence of MI, and its associated mortality, increased similarly among male and female smokers of European countries, as well as Japan.[5, 60] Other studies, by contract, showed a higher RR of MI for female smokers[26] and male smokers.[61] Many prospective studies in Europe and the US provided similar, strong evidence of an excess risk of stroke among male and female smokers,[3, 62-64] but data from Japanese populations are limited and results are not consistent.[6, 8, 9, 13] Many epidemiological and clinical studies of men[2, 19] and some of women [65] in Europe and the US demonstrate a similar increased risk of peptic ulcer in men and women who smoke.[66] However, there have been few Japanese and Asian prospective studies that have examined gender differences on the effects of smoking on peptic ulcer incidence. Our study was unusual in that we examined gender differences on the effects of smoking on several cardiovascular diseases, as well as peptic ulcer disease.

Participants in the present study--atomic bomb survivors and their controls--may not be representative of the general Japanese population, but we believe that the results might be extrapolated to the general population, due to the fact that one third of the participants were minimally exposed (estimated radiation dose, zero), and that the radiation exposure effects were fully accounted for by including radiation dose as a covariate in the analysis. The agreement of our findings on the effects of demographic variables such as age and gender with the findings of others [6, 37] further supports for the validity of our results.

The proportion of men who are current smokers is higher in Japan than in Western countries [9, 44] while the reverse is true for women, although a rise in smoking frequency among young to middle-aged Japanese women since 1990 has been reported.[67] The present results provide further support for smoking cessation as a way to prevent cardiovascular disease and peptic ulcer in Japan.

APPENDIX

International Classification of Diseases Codes			
	ICD edition		
Disease	7th	8th	9th
Myocardial infarction	-	410	410,412
Stroke	330-332,334	430,431,433,434,436	430,431,433, 434,436
Aortic aneurysm	451	441	441
Gastric ulcer	540	531	531
Duodenal ulcer	541	532	532

ACKNOWLEDGMENTS

This publication is based on research performed at the Radiation Effects Research Foundation (RERF), Hiroshima and Nagasaki, Japan. RERF is a private non-profit foundation funded equally by the Japanese Ministry of Health, Labour and Welfare and the US Department of Energy (DOE), the latter through the National Academy of Sciences. This publication was supported by RERF Research Protocol RP 2-75 and in part by a grant from the Japan Arteriosclerosis Prevention Fund.

REFERENCES

[1] Andersen, IB; Jorgensen, T; Bonnevie, O; et al.: Smoking and alcohol intake as risk factors for bleeding and perforated peptic ulcers: a population-based cohort study. *Epidemiology,* 2000, 11, 434-439.

[2] Doll, R; Peto, R; Wheatley, K; et al.: Mortality in relation to smoking: 40 years' observations on male British doctors. *Bmj,* 1994, 309, 901-911.

[3] Wolf, PA; D'Agostino, RB; Kannel, WB; et al.: Cigarette smoking as a risk factor for stroke. The Framingham Study. *Jama,* 1988, 259, 1025-1029.

[4] Hozawa, A; Houston, T; Steffes, MW; et al.: The association of cigarette smoking with self-reported disease before middle age: the Coronary Artery Risk Development in Young Adults (CARDIA) study. *Prev. Med.,* 2006, 42, 193-199.

[5] Nilsson, S; Carstensen, JM; Pershagen, G: Mortality among male and female smokers in Sweden: a 33 year follow up. *J. Epidemiol. Community Health,* 2001, 55, 825-830.

[6] Kiyohara, Y; Ueda, K; Fujishima, M. Smoking and cardiovascular disease in the general population in Japan. *J. Hypertens. Suppl.,* 1990, 8, S9-15.

[7] Tanaka, H; Ueda, Y; Hayashi, M; et al.: Risk factors for cerebral hemorrhage and cerebral infarction in a Japanese rural community.. *Stroke,* 1982, 13, 62-73.

[8] Tanizaki, Y; Kiyohara, Y; Kato, I; et al.: Incidence and risk factors for subtypes of cerebral infarction in a general population: the Hisayama study. *Stroke,* 2000, 31, 2616-2622.

[9] Ueshima, H; Choudhury, SR; Okayama, A; et al.: Cigarette smoking as a risk factor for stroke death in Japan: NIPPON DATA80. *Stroke* 2004, 35, 1836-1841.

[10] Liu, XF; van Melle, G; Bogousslavsky, J. Analysis of risk factors in 3901 patients with stroke. *Chin. Med. Sci. J.,* 2005, 20, 35-39.

[11] Okada, H; Horibe, H; Yoshiyuki, O; et al.: A prospective study of cerebrovascular disease in Japanese rural communities, Akabane and Asahi. Part 1: evaluation of risk factors in the occurrence of cerebral hemorrhage and thrombosis. *Stroke,* 1976, 7, 599-607.

[12] Takeya, Y; Popper, JS; Shimizu, Y et al.: Epidemiologic studies of coronary heart disease and stroke in Japanese men living in Japan, Hawaii and California: incidence of stroke in Japan and Hawaii. *Stroke* 1984, 15, 15-23.

[13] Mannami, T; Iso, H; Baba, S; et al.: Cigarette smoking and risk of stroke and its subtypes among middle-aged Japanese men and women: the JPHC Study Cohort I. *Stroke,* 2004, 35, 1248-1253.

[14] Tokuda, Y. Risk factors for acute myocardial infarction among Okinawans. *J. Nutr. Health Aging* 2005, 9, 272-276.

[15] Okumiya, N; Tanaka, K; Ueda, K; et al.: Coronary atherosclerosis and antecedent risk factors: pathologic and epidemiologic study in Hisayama, Japan. *Am. J. Cardiol.,* 1985, 56, 62-66.

[16] Benfante, R; Yano, K; Hwang, LJ; et al.: Elevated serum cholesterol is a risk factor for both coronary heart disease and thromboembolic stroke in Hawaiian Japanese men. Implications of shared risk. *Stroke* 1994, 25, 814-820.

[17] Yano, K; MacLean, CJ; Reed, DM; et al.: A comparison of the 12-year mortality and predictive factors of coronary heart disease among Japanese men in Japan and Hawaii. *Am. J. Epidemiol.* 1988, 127, 476-487.

[18] Goldberg, RJ; Burchfiel, CM; Benfante, R; et al.: Lifestyle and biologic factors associated with atherosclerotic disease in middle-aged men. 20-year findings from the Honolulu Heart Program. *Arch. Intern. Med.* 1995, 155, 686-694.

[19] Kato, I; Nomura, AM; Stemmermann, GN; et al.: A prospective study of gastric and duodenal ulcer and its relation to smoking, alcohol, and diet. *Am. J. Epidemiol.,* 1992, 135, 521-530.

[20] Wong, FL; Yamada, M; Sasaki, H; et al.: Noncancer disease incidence in the atomic bomb survivors: 1958-1986. *Radiat. Res.,* 1993, 135, 418-430.

[21] Yamada, M; Wong, FL; Fujiwara S et al.: Noncancer disease incidence in atomic bomb survivors, 1958-1998. *Radiat. Res.,* 2004, 161, 622-632.

[22] International Classification of Diseases, 9th Revision (ICD 9). Geneva: WHO; 1977.

[23] Preston, D; Lubin, J; Pierce, D. Epicure User's Guide. Seattle: Hirosoft *International Corp.*; 1993.

[24] Suzuki, K; Kutsuzawa, T; Takita, K; et al.: Clinico-epidemiologic study of stroke in Akita, Japan. *Stroke,* 1987, 18, 402-406.

[25] Rozenthul-Sorokin, N; Ronen, R; Tamir, A; et al.: Stroke in the young in Israel. Incidence and outcomes. *Stroke,* 1996, 27, 838-841.

[26] Prescott, E; Hippe, M; Schnohr, P; et al.: Smoking and risk of myocardial infarction in women and men: longitudinal population study. *Bmj,* 1998, 316, 1043-1047.

[27] Sacco, RL; Benjamin, EJ; Broderick, JP; et al.: American Heart Association Prevention Conference. IV. Prevention and Rehabilitation of Stroke. Risk factors. *Stroke,* 1997, 28, 1507-1517.

[28] Lerner, DJ; Kannel, WB. Patterns of coronary heart disease morbidity and mortality in the sexes: a 26-year follow-up of the Framingham population. *Am. Heart J.,* 1986, 111, 383-390.

[29] Kodama, K; Sasaki, H; Shimizu, Y; Trend of coronary heart disease and its relationship to risk factors in a Japanese population: a 26-year follow-up, Hiroshima/Nagasaki study. *Jpn. Circ. J.,* 1990, 54, 414-421.

[30] Robertson, T; Shimizu, H; Kato, K; et al. Incidence of stroke and coronary heart disease in atomic bomb survivors living in Hiroshima and Nagasaki. 1958-74. Hiroshima: Radiation *Effects Research Foundation*; 1979.

[31] Rodin, MB; Daviglus, ML; Wong, GC; et al.: Middle age cardiovascular risk factors and abdominal aortic aneurysm in older age. *Hypertension,* 2003, 42, 61-68.

[32] Yii, MK. Epidemiology of abdominal aortic aneurysm in an Asian population. *ANZ J. Surg.,* 2003, 73, 393-395.

[33] Hu, YH; Shimizu, H; Kawakami, N; et al.: Increasing trends in mortality rate of aortic aneurysms in Japan, 1955-90. *Tohoku J. Exp. Med.,* 1993, 171, 221-228.

[34] Smoking, lung function and the prognosis of abdominal aortic aneurysm. The UK Small Aneurysm Trial Participants. *Eur. J. Vasc. Endovasc. Surg .,* 2000, 19, 636-642.

[35] Ballaro, A; Cortina-Borja, M; Collin, J. A seasonal variation in the incidence of ruptured abdominal aortic aneurysms. *Eur. J .Vasc. Endovasc. Surg.*, 1998, 15, 429-431.

[36] Kato, I; Tominaga, S; Ito, Y; et al.: Comparative case-control analysis of gastric and duodenal ulcers. *Jpn. J. Public Health,* 1990, 37, 919-925.

[37] Watanabe, Y; Kurata, JH; Kawamoto, K; et al.: Epidemiological study of peptic ulcer disease among Japanese and Koreans in Japan. *J. Clin. Gastroenterol.,* 1992, 15, 68-74.

[38] Friedman, GD; Siegelaub, AB; Seltzer, CC. Cigarettes, alcohol, coffee and peptic ulcer. *N. Engl. J. Med.,* 1974, 290, 469-473.

[39] Sonnenberg, A. Smoking and mortality from peptic ulcer in the United Kingdom. *Gut,* 1986, 27, 1369-1372.

[40] Sonnenberg, A; Everhart, JE: The prevalence of self-reported peptic ulcer in the United States. *Am. J. Public Health,* 1996, 86, 200-205.

[41] Sauvaget, C; Nagano, J; Allen, N; et al.: Intake of animal products and stroke mortality in the Hiroshima/Nagasaki Life Span Study. *Int. J. Epidemiol.,* 2003, 32, 536-543.

[42] Kawachi, I; Colditz, GA; Stampfer, MJ; et al.: Smoking cessation in relation to total mortality rates in women. A prospective cohort study. *Ann. Intern. Med.,* 1993, 119, 992-1000.

[43] Tornwall, ME; Virtamo, J; Haukka, JK; et al.: Life-style factors and risk for abdominal aortic aneurysm in a cohort of Finnish male smokers. *Epidemiology,* 2001, 12, 94-100.

[44] Kawachi, I; Colditz, GA; Stampfer, MJ et al.: Smoking cessation and decreased risk of stroke in women. *Jama,* 1993, 269, 232-236.

[45] Iso, H; Date, C; Yamamoto, A; et al.: Smoking cessation and mortality from cardiovascular disease among Japanese men and women: the JACC Study. *Am. J. Epidemiol.,* 2005, 161, 170-179.

[46] Kawachi, I; Colditz, GA; Stampfer MJ et al.: Smoking cessation and time course of decreased risks of coronary heart disease in middle-aged women. *Arch. Intern. Med.,* 1994, 154, 169-175.

[47] Clavier, I; Hommel, M; Besson, G; et al.: Long-term prognosis of symptomatic lacunar infarcts. A hospital-based study. *Stroke,* 1994, 25, 2005-2009.

[48] Ovbiagele, B; Weir, CJ; Saver, JL; et al.: Effect of smoking status on outcome after acute ischemic stroke. *Cerebrovasc. Dis.,* 2006, 21, 260-265.

[49] Sasaki, H; Wong, FL; Yamada, M; et al.: The effects of aging and radiation exposure on blood pressure levels of atomic bomb survivors. *J. Clin. Epidemiol.,* 2002, 55, 974-981.

[50] Sairenchi, T; Iso, H; Nishimura, A; et al.: Cigarette smoking and risk of type 2 diabetes mellitus among middle-aged and elderly Japanese men and women. *Am. J. Epidemiol.,* 2004, 160, 158-162.

[51] Lederle, FA; Nelson, DB; Joseph, AM: Smokers' relative risk for aortic aneurysm compared with other smoking-related diseases: a systematic review. *J. Vasc. Surg.,* 2003, 38, 329-334.

[52] Johnsen, R; Forde, OH; Straume, B; et al.: Aetiology of peptic ulcer: a prospective population study in Norway. *J. Epidemiol. Community Health,* 1994, 48, 156-160.

[53] Rosenstock, S; Jorgensen, T; Bonnevie, O; et al. Risk factors for peptic ulcer disease: a population based prospective cohort study comprising 2416 Danish adults. *Gut,* 2003, 52, 186-193.

[54] Susser, M. Causes of peptic ulcer. A selective epidemiologic review. *J. Chronic Dis.,* 1967, 20, 435-456.

[55] Graham, DY. Helicobacter pylori: its epidemiology and its role in duodenal ulcer disease. *J. Gastroenterol. Hepatol.* 1991, 6, 105-113.

[56] Asaka, M; Kimura, T; Kudo, M; et al.: Relationship of Helicobacter pylori to serum pepsinogens in an asymptomatic Japanese population.. *Gastroenterology,* 1992, 102, 760-766.

[57] Asaka, M. [Epidemiology of Helicobacter pylori infection in Japan]. *Nippon Rinsho,* 2003, 61, 19-24.

[58] Hakoda, M; Kasagi, F; Kusunoki, Y; et al.: Levels of antibodies to microorganisms implicated in atherosclerosis and of C-reactive protein among atomic bomb survivors. *Radiat. Res*., 2006, 166, 360-366.

[59] Blaser, MJ; Chyou, PH; Nomura, A. Age at establishment of Helicobacter pylori infection and gastric carcinoma, gastric ulcer, and duodenal ulcer risk. *Cancer Res.,* 1995, 55, 562-565.

[60] LaCroix, AZ; Lang, J; Scherr, P; et al.: Smoking and mortality among older men and women in three communities. *N. Engl. J. Med.,* 1991, 324, 1619-1625.

[61] Seltzer, CC. Framingham study data and "established wisdom" about cigarette smoking and coronary heart disease. *J. Clin. Epidemiol.,* 1989, 42, 743-750.

[62] Hart, CL; Hole, DJ; Smith, GD. Comparison of risk factors for stroke incidence and stroke mortality in 20 years of follow-up in men and women in the Renfrew/Paisley Study in Scotland. *Stroke,* 2000, 31, 1893-1896.

[63] Hankey, GJ. Smoking and risk of stroke. *J Cardiovasc Risk*, 1999, 6, 207-211.

[64] Shinton, R; Beevers, G. Meta-analysis of relation between cigarette smoking and stroke. *Bmj,* 1989, 298, 789-794.

[65] Anda, RF; Williamson, DF; Escobedo LG et al.: Smoking and the risk of peptic ulcer disease among women in the United States. *Arch. Intern. Med.* 1990, 150, 1437-1441.

[66] Ashley, MJ. Smoking and diseases of the gastrointestinal system: an epidemiological review with special reference to sex differences. *Can. J. Gastroenterol* ., 1997, 11, 345-352.

[67] Ministry of Health, Labor and Welfare.. Tobacco or Health. Cited 2007 July 6 available from hrrp://www.health-net.or.jp/tobacco/product/ pd090000.html.

In: Ulcers: Causes, Diagnosis, and Treatment ISBN: 978-1-60741-253-3
Editors: Danijel Erceg et al. pp. 65-69

Chapter 5

ANTISECRETORY COMPOUNDS AND STRESS-INDUCED GASTRIC ULCERS

S. Evangelista[*]
Menarini Ricerche SpA, Preclinical Development, Florence, Italy

ABSTRACT

Acute gastric mucosal lesions, which can develop within a few hours after polytrauma, shock, major operations, central nervous system lesions, or severe infection, cause about one third of the cases of gastrointestinal bleeding. We analyzed and compared the effectiveness of two antisecretory compounds such as cimetidine and omeprazole on acute gastric mucosal lesions and acidity induced by stress in rats. Male Sprague-Dawley rats after 24 h fasting, received omeprazole (2.9–29 μmol/kg p.o.), cimetidine (99–396 μmol/kg p.o.) or their respective vehicle 1 h before being exposed to water immersion stress for 3 h. All rats were ulcer-indexed according to the length and number of their ulcers. The stomach contents were aspirated for acid output and pH analysis. Omeprazole was more effective than cimetidine in keeping gastric pH high and lowering the total gastric acid output. Macroscopical examination of acute gastric mucosal erosions showed that omeprazole was 10 times more effective than cimetidine on molar basis in the inhibition of ulcer formation. The sudden increase in pH afforded by

[*] Correspondence Address: Menarini Ricerche SpA, Via Sette Santi 1, 50131 Florence, Italy Tel: int+055/5680519, Fax: int+055/5680510, e-mail: sevangelista@menarini-ricerche.it

proton pump inhibitors indicate them as first-line therapy for treatment and prophylaxis of stress ulcer patients.

A recent survey performed on two thousand critical care physicians has indicated that respiratory failure, shock/hypotension, sepsis and major head injury/neurologic insult are the most frequent reasons associated with gastric stress ulcers in humans [1]. Antisecretory compounds are the most used therapy for this kind of damage [2, 3], being able, e.g., to reduce mortality and re-bleeding in patients with high-risk endoscopic findings. We have compared a proton pump inhibitor such as omeprazole with an H-2 receptor antagonist such as cimetidine in an experimental model of stress ulcers.

Male albino rats, Sprague-Dawley Nossan strain, weighing 180–210 g, were housed at constant room temperature (21±1°C), relative humidity (60 %) and with 12 h light-dark cycle (light on at 6.00 a.m.). Gastric ulcers were induced in 24-h-fasted rats by water immersion stress (WIS): the animals were individually placed in a plexigass cylinder (40 cm height, 18 cm internal diameter) containing water (15 cm depth) maintained at 25 ± 1°C for a period of 3 h. Oral omeprazole (2.9–29 μmol/kg) or cimetidine (99–396 μmol/kg) were administered to the animals 60 min before the WIS procedure. The animals were sacrificed by cervical dislocation 3 h after WIS, their gastric ulcers measured, by an observer unaware of the treatments, by means of a binocular microscope (magnification x10) to determine the lesion index. Lesions smaller than 1 mm were assigned a rating of 1, lesions measuring 1–2 mm were assigned a rating of 2 and lesions measuring more than 2 mm were given a rating according to their length in mm. The overall total was designated the "lesion index" according to Holzer et al. [4].

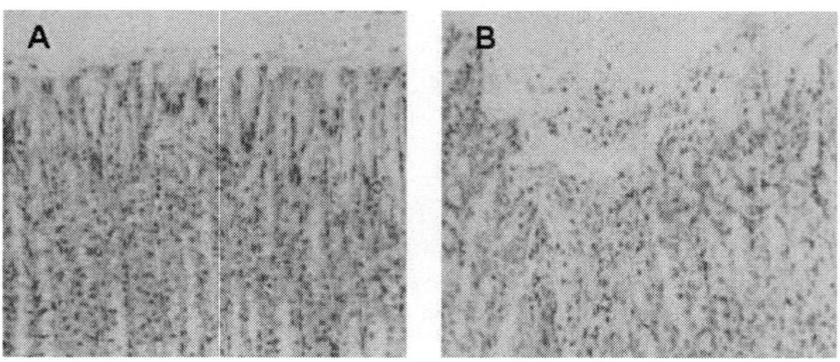

Figure 1. Histological appearance of intact gastric mucosa (A) and erosion induced by water immersion stress in the oxyntic mucosa (B). Haematoxylin and eosin stain, magnification x 200, modified from Warzecha et al. (2001).

Table 1. Effect of omeprazole and cimetidine on gastric acidity and ulcers induced by water immersion stress (WIS).

Treatments (μmol/kg p.o.)	pH	meq H^+/ml	Ulcer number	Ulcer index
Control	4.87±0.31	0.75±0.30		
WIS	4.15±0.21	1.04±0.38	16.1±2.9	26.2±5.1
WIS+Omeprazole 2.9	4.16±0.13	0.61±0.09*	15.8±2.1	27.8±6.8
WIS+Omeprazole 14.5	4.74±0.28	0.41±0.26**	11.4±3.6*	14.6±4.2*
WIS+Omeprazole 29	5.11±0.60	0.32±0.13**	4.6±2.6**	6.2±4.2**
WIS+Cimetidine 99	4.30±0.30	0.89±0.27	8.4±2.2*	25.8±6.8
WIS+Cimetidine 198	4.08±0.27	0.44±0.07 **	9.6±3.6*	15.0±7.0*
WIS+Cimetidine 396	3.92±0.22	0.49±0.11**	3.8±1.7**	3.0±1.4**

*=p<0.05 and **=p<0.01 vs WIS

Intragastric acidity was determined by washing the stomach with 10 ml of distilled water. The samples were centrifuged and the acid supernatant was titrated to pH 7 by an automatic pH meter.

Statistical analysis was performed by means of analysis of variance followed by Tukey's test. All data were expressed as mean ± S.E.

WIS produced punctiform or linear lesions that were randomly distributed over the glandular mucosa. The lesions were characterized histologically by an infilatrate of erytrocytes, sheets of mucosal layers in the lumen, necrosis of the superficial layers and oedema of the submucosa (Figure 1).

As shown in Table 1, WIS induced a 38 % increase in gastric acidity without influencing significatively the luminal gastric pH.

Omeprazole (2.9–29 μmol/kg p.o.) dose-dependently reduced the number and index of the lesions induced by WIS as well as gastric acidity that was inhibited by 69 % at the highest dose (Table 1). Increasing doses of omeprazole produced a trend of an increased luminal pH (Table 1). Likewise cimetidine (99–396 μmol/kg p.o.) reduced WIS induced ulcers but was less active in reducing gastric acidity and did not affect the luminal pH (Table 1). Macroscopical examination of the number of gastric ulcers induced by WIS showed that omeprazole was 10 times more effective than cimetidine on a molar basis in the ulcer prevention (ED_{50} were 20.3 vs 210 μmol/kg, for omeprazole and cimetidine, respectively). Similarly, in immobilization stress induced erosions in rats, the antiulcer effect of omeprazole given i.v. was found superior to that afforded by famotidine, another H-2 receptor antagonist [5].

The mechanisms considered to play a role in the pathogenesis of water immersion stress induced gastric lesions in rats are the increase in gastric acid and pepsin secretion, decrease in blood flow and bicarbonate secretion, suppression of mucosal generation of prostaglandins, inhibition of mucosal growth and cell proliferation and alteration of gastric motility [6, 7]. Both H-2 receptor antagonists and proton pump inhibitors did not affect blood flow and altered gastric motility [7, 8] at least at the doses utilized in these experiments and therefore their beneficial effects are mainly due to their antisecretory activity. The rapidity by which omeprazole is able to increase the pH and to decrease the gastric acidity play a role in the prevention of ulcer erosions induced by stress as found in other experimental models of gastric ulcers such as those induced by nonsteroidal anti-inflammatory drugs [9]. Clinical trials have clearly shown that maintaining an intragastric pH above 4.5–6 can prevent injury and that a pH below 4 increased the risk of stress ulceration [10]. Due to their long-lasting inhibition of gastric secretion, proton pump inhibitors can be considered the first choice class of drug for stress ulcers and recent studies have indicated that for their pharmacodynamic characteristics these drugs can be given by frequent oral routes in order to replace the recommended but cost-expensive intravenous bolus plus infusion administration [11].

REFERENCES

[1] Daley, RJ; Rebuck, JA; Welage, LS; Rogers, FS. Prevention of stress ulceration: current trends in critical care. *Crit Care Med,* 2004, 32, 2008-2013.

[2] Levy, MJ; Seelling, CB; Robinson, NJ; Ranney, JE. Comparison of omeprazole and ranitidine for stress ulcer prophylaxis. *Dig Dis Sci,* 1997, 42, 1255-1259.

[3] Leontiadis, GI; Sreedharan, A; Dorward, S; Barton, P; Delaney, B; Howden, CW; et al., Systematic reviews of the clinical effectiveness and cost-effectiveness of proton pump inhibitors in acute upper gastrointestinal bleeding. *Health Technol Assess,* 2007, 11, 1-164.

[4] Holzer, P; Lippe, IT. Stimulation of afferent nerve endings by intragastric capsaicin protects against ethanol-induced damage of gastric mucosa. *Neuroscience,* 1988, 27, 981-987.

[5] Topaloglu, U; Muftuoglu, T; Akturk, Z; Ekinci, H; Peker, O; Unalmiser, S. Omeprazole is more effective than famotidine for preventing acute gastritis in rats. *Surg Today,* 2004, 34, 690-694.

[6] Kitagawa, H; Fujiwara, M; Osumi, Y. Effect of water immersion stress on gastric secretion and mucosal blood flow in rats. *Gastroenterology,* 1979, 14, 298-302.

[7] Warzecha, Z; Dembinski, A; Brzozowski, T; Ceranowicz, P; Dembinski, M; Stachura, J; et al., Histamine in stress ulcer prophylaxis in rats. *J Physiol Pharmacol,* 2001, 52, 407-421.

[8] Yamamoto, O; Okada, Y; Okabe, S. Effects of proton pump inhibitor, omeprazole on gastric secretion and gastric and duodenal ulcers or erosions in rats. *Dig Dis Sci,* 1984, 29, 394-401.

[9] Evangelista, S. Increase in pH and prevention of gastropathy induced by nonsteroidal anti-inflammatory drugs. Scand J Gastroenterol, 1997, 32, 1071.

[10] Stollman, N; Metz, DC. Pathophysiology and prophylaxis of stress ulcer in intensive care unit patients. *J Crit Care,* 2005, 20, 35-45.

[11] Laine, L; Shah, A; Bemanian, S. Intragastric pH with oral vs intravenous bolus plus infusion proton pump inhibitor therapy in patients with bleeding ulcers. *Gastroenterology*, 2008, 134, 1836-1841.

In: Ulcers: Causes, Diagnosis, and Treatment ISBN: 978-1-60741-253-3
Editors: Danijel Erceg et al. pp. 71-88

Chapter 6

ATYPICAL SKIN ULCERS

***Jochanan E. Naschitz*[1] *and Akiva Trattner*[2]**
[1]Flieman Hopsital, Haifa, Israel
[2] Tel Aviv University, Tel Aviv, Israel

It is hyaluronate which stabilizes the intercellular structures of the skin by forming a viscoelastic network in which collagen and elastin fibers are embedded. With aging, the hyaluronate in the extracellular matrix is diminished, leading to easy tearing and lacerations. The term 'dermatoporosis' has been proposed to embrace the different manifestations and implications of the skin atrophy, cutaneous fragility and insufficiency syndrome that is related to aging. The clinical manifestations of dermatoporosis usually become apparent after the age 60 years; more advanced dermatoporosis is perceived at 70 to 90 years of age. The dermatoporosis syndrome comprises: skin atrophy, senile purpura, stellate pseudoscars, frequent skin laceration, delayed wound healing and subcutaneous bleeding. On skin ultrasonography, the dermatoporotic skin is characterized by diminished thickness of the epidermis and dermis. Microscopic examination of skin biopsy specimen shows thinning of the epidermis and dermis the rete ridges being lost, as well as diminished collagen fibers, elastic fibers and mucin content in the dermis [1,2]. Dermatoporosis may be primarily related to the aging process, in which genetic factors may play a significant role [1], or may be secondary to chronic corticosteroid treatment either topical or following systemic administration. The primary and iatrogenic dermatoporosis have similar appearance on physical examination [3].

Skin atrophy is seen mainly in the areas exposed to sun, which are the posterior surfaces of the forearms and the pretibial zones. The atrophic skin becomes thin, transparent, with numerous wrinkles, and often purpura and pseudoscars. Senile purpura results from minimal trauma and in the absence of a coagulation disorder. Moreover, large hematomas may accrue after minimal trauma within the virtual space between the dermis and subcutaneous adipose tissue or between the subcutaneous adipose tissue and muscle fascia. Dermatoporosis may be complicated by *non-healing skin ulcers*. The mechanisms responsible for delayed wound healing of the dermatoporotic skin are decreased proliferative capacity of keratinocytes and fibroblasts, abundant production of matrix metalloproteinases and secretion of cytokines which inhibit the dedifferentiation of keratinocytes [4,5]. Dermatoporosis should be treated to prevent pending complications [1,2].

I. Skin Ulcers in the Elderly – Four Common Etiologies

Four etiologies account for the large majority of skin ulcers in the elderly: ischemia, venous insufficiency, neuropathy and trauma [6-10].

Ulcers due to arterial insufficiency typically occur on the toes, heels or anterior shin. Arterial ulcers are round or punched-out and well demarcated; their base is covered by a yellow fibrin layer or by a necrotic eschar; tendons or bone may be exposed. Peripheral obstructive arterial disease is a common cause of ischemic ulcers; the patients complain of intermittent claudication and ischemic rest pain; chronic limb ischemia is characterized by hair loss, skin atrophy, nail dystrophy, and decreased or not palpable pulses; the ankle-brachial index (the ankle-to brachial systolic blood pressure ratio) is usually <0.7.

Venous ulcerations typically occur above the lateral or medial malleoli, but infection or trauma may localize the venous ulcers to other sites. Venous ulcers are usually shallow, have irregular borders, their base may be fibrinous or covered by granulation tissue. The patients usually have a history of venous insufficiency or deep venous thrombosis. On physical examination there are varicous veins, leg edema, hyperpigmentation, stasis dermatitis or lipodermatosclerosis. The ankle-brachial index is usually >0.9 (normal). It is often stated that clinical examination of the patient in good light provides nearly all the information necessary for the diagnosis of chronic venous insufficiency. However, the predictive value of clinical indicators of venous disease did not exceed 0.76 in one study [11]. To increase the accuracy of diagnosis of venous ulcer, clinical examination should be combined with non-invasive hemodynamic assessment of the venous circulation.

Neuropathic ulcers occur at pressure points, i.e. under metatarsal heads, over toe joints, under the heel, on the inner side of the first metatarsal head, and over the maleoli. The patients often complain of foot numbness or burning. Sensory neuropathy often leads to a loss of the protective sensation. Motor neuropathy leads to small muscle wasting and, consequently, to imbalance between flexors and extensors of the lower limb causing clawing of toes and prominence of the metatarsal heads that are thus exposed to pressure. Sympathetic autonomic neuropathy leads to dry, cracked, and fissured skin over the lower leg. Neuropathic ulcers are characterized by blister hemorrhage, necrosis, callus surrounding the wound, and exposure of underlying structures. Claw toes and Charcot joints may be associated findings. On monofilament testing for light touch sensitivity, the inability to perceive a 10 *g* of force applied by the monofilament is related to clinically significant large-fiber neuropathy [12]. The ankle brachial index is normal, unless neuropathy is associated with peripheral arterial insufficiency. Neuropathy may coexist with ischemia and act synergistically in increasing the risk of skin laceration, necrosis and defective wound heeling. Diabetics are prone to develop neuropathic ulcers. Rarer conditions responsible for neuropathic ulcers include chronic alcoholism with malnutrition, leprosy, tabes dorsalis, spina bifida, and syringomyelia.

Among traumatic skin ulcers, pressure ulcers are defined as areas of localized damage to the skin and underlying tissue caused by pressure, shear, friction, or a combination of these [13]. The National Pressure Ulcer Advisory Panel in 1989 distinguishes four stages of pressure ulcers depending on the level of tissue breakdown: stage I characterized by nonblanching erythema of intact skin; stage II characterized by partial-thickness skin loss involving the epidermis, dermis, or both; stage III characterized by full-thickness skin loss involving damage or necrosis to subcutaneous tissue, which may extend down to underlying fascia; stage IV characterized by full-thickness skin loss with extensive destruction, tissue necrosis, or damage to muscle or bone. Pressure ulcers usually develop on the lower half of the body, two thirds around the pelvis and a third on the lower limbs, with heel ulceration being most common. Risk factors for pressure ulceration are chronic disease, cerebrovascular accident, impaired nutrition, confinement to chair or bed, faecal incontinence, fractured neck of femur, altered consciousness, limited mobility, sensory impairment, severe chronic or terminal disease, vascular disease, malnutrition and dehydration [14].

The assessment and management of ischemic, venous, neuropathic ulcers and pressure sores has been reviewed in the recent literature and guidelines for treatment have been proposed [13-30]. Essentials are briefly reminded now.

Microbiology of Chronic Wounds

The significance of positive bacteriology smears and cultures differs when taken from neuropathic, venous or arterial leg ulcers. Only 22% of the venous ulcers with a positive smear developed a clinical infection; this contrasts to 70% of the arterial and diabetic ulcers where positive smears were indicative of clinical infection [22]. Therefore, wound smears should not be obtained routinely from patients with chronic venous ulcers. In 90% of diabetic skin ulcers that did not extend to the bone, the swab cultures identified all micro-organisms that were isolated from the deep tissue biopsy specimen [21]. Therefore, wound smears should be obtained routinely from patients with diabetic ulcers. Yet, preference is given to cultures obtained by curettage following debridement in order to identify the causative organisms in diabetic ulcers as well in other chronic wounds.

Basically, assessment of chronic wounds for the presence of infection is a difficult task. The distinction between bacterial colonization and infection cannot be founded on bacteriology alone, but relies very much on clinical judgment [20].

Likelihood of Osteomyelitis Adjacent to a Chronic Wound

The likelihood of osteomyelitis in a diabetic patient presenting a lower extremity ulcer can be estimated based on three criteria [25]. First, an ulcer area larger than 2 cm^2 indicates a 56% likelihood of osteomyelitis. Second, a positive probe-to-bone test indicates osteomyelitis with 53% probability. The probe-to-bone test is performed with a sterile, blunt, stainless steel probe. The examiner gently probes the wound for the presence of a rock-hard structure at the wound base. A 'positive probe-to-bone result' indicates that the necrotic process probably involves the bone. Third, an ESR greater than 70 mm/h is associated with a 66% probability of osteomyelitis. Most clinicians believe that the presence of these 3 variables together would make the diagnosis of osteomyelitis certain and would treat as osteomyelitis [25].

Other clinicians might choose to order an MRI examination. A positive MRI result in combination with any one of the three clinical variables increases the probability of osteomyelitis to greater than 80%. On the other hand, the body temperature, ulcer inflammation, white blood cell count, and swab culture do not appear to be helpful in establishing the diagnosis of osteomyelitis in patients with diabetes and a lower extremity ulcer.

Prevention of Pressure Ulcers

Although a number of randomized controlled trials have evaluated preventive strategies for pressure ulcers, many of them had important methodological limitations [15]. Frequent change in body position is a mainstay in pressure ulcer prevention protocols, but there is insufficient evidence to recommend specific turning regimens for patients with impaired mobility [13,15]. Current practice requires that any individual at risk for developing pressure ulcers should be repositioned when lying in the bed at least every 2 hours; for patients who are in a chair repositioning should be done every hour. Pressure-relieving mattresses are classified into three groups, and patients must meet clinical criteria before reimbursement is provided: group 1 (static overlays and replacement mattresses); group 2 (low-air-loss beds, alternating pressure, and powered or nonpowered overlays or mattresses); and group 3 (air-fluidized beds). Most pressure-relieving mattresses do not decrease pressure below capillary closing pressure of 32 mm Hg; therefore patients need repositioning every 2 hours. The only true pressure-relieving surface is the air-fluidized bed, which is used for patients after flap surgeries and for patients who have no turning surfaces. In sitting position, there are specialty cushions that also reduce pressure and help to decrease the risk of pressure ulcers.

Treatment of Pressure Ulcers [13-15,31,32]

Making an accurate bacteriologic diagnosis of pressure ulcers is difficult, since every wound is contaminated by bacteria but not all wounds are infected. Swabbing a pressure ulcer often yields organisms that are colonizers and not actually causes of infection. It may be most appropriate to aspirate material from the margin or base of the pressure ulcer, directing the needle through intact skin or take a tissue biopsy. 'Critical colonization' is defined by bacterial load exceeding 1×10^5 colonies/g of tissue. Critical colonization affects the body's ability to heal and it becomes necessary to treat as infection. Clinical signs of infection are increased drainage, odor, surrounding erythema, pain, warmth, or simply a wound that has failed to improve despite adequate removal of necrotic tissue and maintenance of a moist wound environment. The time frame is usually a lack of progression after 14 days of therapy.

A consensus panel recommended the following wound dressings for the management of chronic wounds: in the debridement stage - hydrogels; for hemorrhagic wounds - alginates; for malodorous wounds - activated charcoal; in the granulation stage - foam and low-adherence dressings; in the epithelialization stage - hydrocolloid and low-adherence dressings [31]. Topical therapies for infected wounds include silver dressings, cadexomer iodine, hydrogen peroxide, povidone-iodine, diluted sodium hypochlorite solution, and chlorpactin. None of these treatments should be used longer than 14 days, because they can be toxic to healthy tissues. Topical antimicrobial agents have not been shown to be effective.

There is no need to treat a pressure ulcer with systemic antibiotics unless there are signs of adjacent cellulitis or osteomyelitis. Pressure ulcer–associated cellulitis, osteomyelitis, or bacteremia are usually caused by *P. mirabilis, S. aureus,* or *B. fragilis.* In general, any regimen that is active against the majority of organisms that are usually causal is appropriate. Although a 10- to 14-day course is commonly prescribed, there is no evidence based data to support this recommendation. A chronic, indolent, non-healing wound may reflect the development of underlying osteomyelitis, the flora of which is often Gram negative or anaerobic. Antibiotics are often started empirically. Osteomyelitis requires a more extended course of therapy. In patients with nutritional impairments, dietary supplements may be beneficial. Rarely, amyloidosis or malignancy may arise as a result of chronic pressure ulceration.

Treatment of Venous Ulcers [19]

Venous ulcer healing is facilitated by applying adequate compression to the lower extremity. The use of a class 3 high-compression therapy (three layer or four layer, low stretch or paste-containing bandages, e.g., Unna's boot) is indicated in the treatment of venous ulcers. The degree of compression must be modified when mixed venous/arterial disease is diagnosed on diagnostic work-up. The ankle brachial index is an important factor to consider in determining compression appropriateness. The type of dressing applied beneath compression has not been shown to affect ulcer healing [16,17]. Necrotic or devitalized tissue (tissue that is laden with bacteria) should be removed. If infection is suspected in a debrided ulcer, or if epithelialization from the margin is not progressing within 2 weeks of debridement and compression therapy, cultures should be performed on aerobic and anaerobic media by tissue biopsy or by a validated quantitative swab technique. Antibacterial preparations should only be used in cases of defined infection and not for bacterial colonization [23]. Topically applied antimicrobials can be effective. For ulcers with $\geq 1 \times 10^6$ colony forming units/g of tissue or any tissue level of beta hemolytic streptococci following adequate debridement, topical antimicrobial therapy in indicated to decrease the bacterial level. Cellulitis surrounding the venous ulcer should be treated with systemic gram-positive bactericidal antibiotics.

Superficial venous surgery is associated with similar rates of ulcer healing to compression alone, but with less recurrence. The effect of deep venous insufficiency on the efficacy of surgery is unclear [18]. A significant proportion of patients are unsuitable for surgical treatment. Growth factors, grafting, biologic skin substitutes, dressings, and oral medication have differing levels of evidence supporting their use [33].

Leg ulcers that worsen in size and symptoms despite treatment, or do not show any improvement over four weeks of treatment, should raise suspicion that the ulcer etiology is not venous in origin or that the therapy needs to be re-evaluated. At this point, specific cultures for mycobacteria and/or fungi are useful, as well as biopsies for histology.

Treatment of Diabetic Foot Ulcers [34]

Local treatment of the ulcer consists of repeated debridement and dressing, though the evidence of benefit of surgical debridement is not strong. Two studies reported a significant benefit of debridement with larvae. Complete excision of plantar neuropathic ulcers is associated with faster wound healing and with fewer recurrences. Some evidence was found to support hydrogels as desloughing agents. Systemic hyperbaric oxygen may be beneficial and decrease the need for major amputations; there are sufficient data to justify its use especially when revascularization is not possible [34,35]. The benefit of topically administered hyperbaric oxygen is not established.

Whether topical negative pressure may promote healing of post-operative wounds is subject to controversy [36,37]. There is currently little evidence to suggest that growth factors and other agents modulating aspects of wound biology should be adopted in routine practice. Bioengineered skin products and skin grafts are widely used in some institutions, but their benefit has not been clearly established.

II. Other Etiologies of Skin Ulcers

In addition to the above described and frequently met skin ulcers, a variety of uncommon or rare etiologies should be considered in the differential diagnosis [30,38-44], as follows:

A. Ischemic ulcers may complicate the course of thrombangiitis obliterans, vasculitis (in particular microscopical variant polyangiitis nodosa, cryoglobuninemia, rheumatoid arthritis, Wegener's granulomatosis, systemic lupus erythematosus, nodular vasculitis), cholesterol embolism, antiphospholipid antibody syndrome, and calciphylaxis.

B. *Hematological disorders:* sickle cell anemia, warfarin-induced skin necrosis, heparin-induced thrombocytopenia, disseminated intravascular coagulation, essential thrombocythemia, therapy with hydroxyurea.

C. *Trauma:* burns, cold, factitial, stings, bites, skin aging.

D. Metabolic disorders: diabetes mellitus (necrobiosis lipoidica diabeticorum), gout.

E. *Infections:* ecthyma gangrenosum, furuncle, mycobacteria (Burundi ulcer caused by Mycobacterium ulcerans, erythema induratum Bazin caused by Mycobacterium tuberculosis), septic emboli, cutaneous leishmaniasis, cutaneous antrax, syphilis, leprosy, fungal infection (trichophytin granuloma, Cryptococcus neofomans, Coccidioides immitis).

F. *Neoplasia:* cutaneous T cell lymphoma, basal cell carcinoma, metastatic tumors, Kaposi sarcoma, squamous cell carcinoma, Merkel cell tumor, malignant transformation of a benign ulcer or scar ('Marjolin's ulcer').

G. *Panniculitis:* Weber Christian disease, pancreatic fat necrosis, alpha1-antitripsin deficiency.

H. *Neutrophilic dermatoses:* pyoderma gangrenosum, Sweet's syndrome.

Chronic leg ulceration is often met in patients during a hospital admission for various causes. Regardless of cause, hospital admission represents an opportunity for full examination of ulcers and further investigations or specialist referral if needed. Knowledge of different patterns of skin ulcers is important, to alert physicians to atypical appearances and lead to appropriate investigations and treatment [44-46]. Making a definite diagnosis is important for tailoring the treatment: corticosteroids for pyoderma gangrenosum or idiopathic vasculitides, antiviral treatment for hepatitis C virus-associated mixed cryoglobulinemia, antimicrobial or antifungal agents for specific infections, treatments for metabolic, hematological and neoplastic disorders.

III. Case History

The diagnosis may indeed be challenging, as illustrated in the following case history.

Case 1 – echymoses, crusts and skin ulcer A 72-yr-old woman has been suffering from progressive disability due to heart failure and chronic obstructive pulmonary disease. A recent exacerbation with pulmonary edema and atrial fibrillation with fast ventricular response was the cause of her admission to the medical ward. She was treated with furosemide, enalapril, pravastatin, verapamil, alopurinol and warfarin. A course of prednisone was instituted for exacerbation of chronic obstructive pulmonary disease, initially 40 mg/day than tapered to 20 mg/day; ciprofloxacin was added. On echocardiography, there were findings consistent severe pulmonary hypertension, mild aortic regurgitation, mild mitral stenosis and regurgitation, the left atrium diameter was 48 mm, and the left ventricular contractility was preserved. The patient had recently discontinued smoking. She was dwelling in the community, not being severely limited in activities of daily living.

Ten days later the patient was transferred to our geriatric ward for aftercare and rehabilitation. At this time she was receiving furosemide 120 mg, enalapril 20 mg, pravastatin 20 mg, verapamil 120 mg, alopurinol 100 mg, prednisone 20 mg, warfarin 2.5 mg, and ciprofloxacin 1 g/day. On physical examination the patient was confused, the bodily temperature was 36.8^{o}C, the blood pressure 120/72 mmHg, the heart rate 86 bpm, the respiratory rate 32 /min, the arterial oxygen saturation was 76% while breathing ambient air 93% on nasal oxygen mask. The jugular veins were engorged. The thorax showed barrel type deformity. Dry crackles were perceived over the lower half of the lung fields and a grade 4/6 systolic murmur at the cardiac apex and aortic foci. The skin in the distal area on the calves showed a mix of brown and violet shades; in the hyperpigmented areas the skin and subcutaneous tissues were indurated. Fourteen shallow skin lesions were counted, spreading over the distal part of the left thigh and left calf; these lesions measured 0.5 – 1 cm in diameter, were well demarcated, roundish, with slightly irregular borders; the lesions were covered by brownish crusts of apparently different ages. Laboratory tests were remarkable for C reactive protein 30 mg/L, serum creatinine 1.6 mg/dL, albumin 3.3 g/L, PT-INR 2.4, activated partial prothrombin time 32 seconds. Results of the blood cell count, liver function tests and urinalysis were within the normal range. Chest X-rays showed an alveolar infiltrate confined to the lower lobe of the left lung.

The patient's previous medications were continued except for ciprofloxacine that was replaced by piperacilline-tazobactam 4.5g x3/day intravenously, and oxygen administered continuously by nasal mask. The disease course was complicated by a succession of events: delirium, that remitted after tapering the dose of prednisone to 5 mg/day; watery diarrhea clostridium toxin negative, which remitted on oral metronidazol treatment; a difficult to achieve warfarin therapeutic goal (PT-INR was in the range 1.3 to 1.7); and two echymoses emerging on the extensor aspect of the patient's left forearm, which subsequently became hemorrhagic blisters, expanding over one week time.

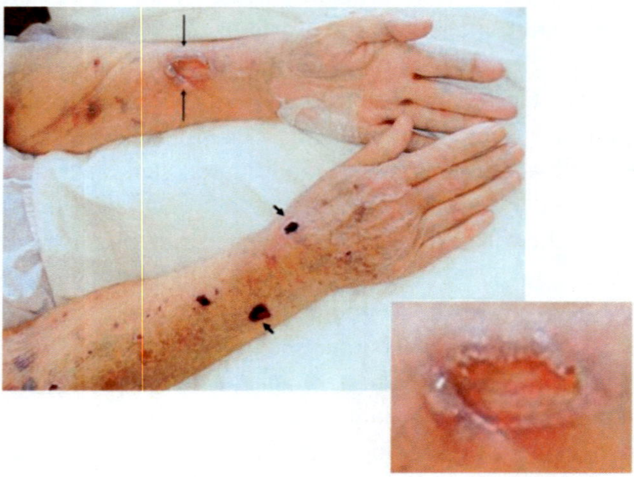

Figure 1. A skin ulcer is seen on the volar aspect of the left forearm (thin arrows). A magnification of the ulcerated area is shown in the inset. About 10 cm proximal to the ulcer there is a scaling crust surrounded by echymosis. The latter two lesions represent different outcomes of hemorrhagic blisters, which preceded by 7-10 days to the present findings. Numerous small lesions covered by brownish-violet crusts are seen on the dorsal aspect of the right forearm (thick arrows).

The larger of the two blisters reached 5 cm in diameter, had peripheral red borders and a violaceous liquid center. The nature of these skin lesions, blisters as well as areas covered by crusts, was unclear; a dermatologist consultant recommended that lesional skin biopsies be taken. Skin punch biopsies were obtained from the peripheral rim of the larger lesion. The content of the blister was aspirated and grew methicillin-resistant Staphylococcus aureus. Treatment with vancomycin was administered intravenously and hydrogel dressings were applied locally. A few days later, the lesion had transformed into a well demarcated ulcer with violaceous undermined borders and a clean basis (Figure 1). The skin biopsy showed an uncharacteristic mixed cellular infiltrate in the epidermis, dermis and subcutaneous layers.

The differential diagnosis of the patient's skin lesions addressed several dermatologic disorders as well as cutaneous manifestations of systemic diseases and iatrogenic effects of corticosteroids and warfarin treatment. A 'pattern diagnosis' was attempted based on the appearance of the smaller skin lesions (that went through evolutionary stages of shallow skin necrosis covered by a crust) and the larger lesion (that went through evolutionary stages of a hemorrhagic blister to deep skin ulcer). The latter lesion was reminiscent of pyoderma gangrenosum.

Pyoderma Gangrenosum

The two primary variants of pyoderma gangrenosum are the classic ulcerative form usually occurring on the legs, and the more superficial variant known as atypical pyoderma gangrenosum that often occurs on the hands. Pyoderma gangrenosum may occur as a primary disorder or in association with another disorder, most often ulcerative colitis, regional enteritis, leukemia, preleukemic states or monoclonal gammopathies [48,49]. In addition to involvement of the skin, other organ systems may be affected in pyoderma gangrenosum by sterile neutrophilic micro-abscesses, which may localize to the lungs, heart, central nervous system, gastrointestinal tract, eyes, liver, spleen, bones or lymph nodes. Systemic manifestations are seen in 50% of patients with pyoderma gangrenosum; they can occur prior to, concurrently or following the cutaneous manifestations of the disease.

Patients with pyoderma gangrenosum usually describe the initial lesion as a small, red papule or pustule changing into a larger ulcerative lesion. Lesions may occur singly or in groups, most commonly on the lower limbs, although they may appear anywhere on the body. The lesions have a liquefying centre without eschar formation, purple undermining borders, which may be covered by hemorrhagic blisters. Pathergy, the phenomenon whereby lesions of a disease can be induced at sites of skin trauma, occurs in up to 50% of patients [48]. Pain is a frequent complaint of patients with pyoderma gangrenosum (pain was not present in our patient).

The histopathologic findings in pyoderma gangrenosum are not specific. Nevertheless, taking a biopsy is recommended in almost all affected patients because its usefulness in excluding other diseases. Microscopic features of pyoderma gangrenosum are massive neutrophilic infiltration associated with hemorrhage and necrosis of the overlying epidermis. Neutrophils may be observed around and within the vessel walls but the full picture of vasculitis is usually absent. The microscopical findings may simulate an abscess or cellulitis. In early disease, a mixed cellular infiltrate may be present [48]. In view of the nonspecific features on histological examination, the diagnosis of pyoderma gangrenosum rests on clinical and pathologic features and also on exclusion of various conditions that may cause skin ulcers [48].

Therapy of pyoderma gangrenosum is based on corticosteroids and immunosuppressants. The smaller early lesions may be treated with intra-lesional injection of triamcinolone. Administration of systemic corticosteroids is recommended for larger active or fully evolved lesions. Prednisone 40 to 80 mg daily is required for initial control of the disease, followed by later tapering of the dosage. Pyoderma gangrenosum patients required a mean 11.5 +/- 11.1 months of treatment to achieve remission compared with 9.0 +/- 13.7 months for patients with atypical pyoderma gangrenosum [48]. Wound dressings are useful to minimize pain and the risk of secondary infection. The application of topical antibacterials is not recommended, but systemic antibacterial therapy is mandatory when infection is present. Recurrences are frequent after treatment termination [49-51].

Overall, the appearance of the patient's larger lesion was consistent with the superficial variant of pyoderma gangrenosum known as atypical pyoderma gangrenosum, provided all other etiologies of skin ulceration could be excluded. The numerous minute lesions on the patient's extremities but sparing the trunk could be explained as manifestations of pathergy. There were, however, several inconsistencies with this diagnosis. First, the skin lesions had appeared while the patient was receiving prednisone, initially 40 mg and later 20 mg/day. The initial presentation of pyoderma gangrenosum under pharmacologic dose prednisone treatment is uncommon. Later in the course of hospitalization, under the impression that prednisone might be the cause of the patient's confusional state, the dose was tapered to 5 mg/day. The delirium remitted and at the same time the skin lesions improved. The relatively fast improvement under physiological doses of corticosteroid administration is also uncharacteristic for pyoderma gangrenosum. Pyoderma gangrenosum being a diagnosis by exclusion, other entities were listed in the differential diagnosis.

Easily excluded based on clinical findings, histology and results of laboratory tests was a spectrum of ischemic ulcers, vasculitides, infectious ulcers (ecthyma gangrenosum, furuncle, mycobacterial and fungal ulcers), and ulcerated neoplasms.

Dissecting hematoma of the skin is a complication due to mechanical fragility of the aged skin. It occurs predominantly in the lower extremities of elderly patients suffering from skin aging (dermatoporosis). There is a female predisposition to dermatoporosis in general and dissecting hematoma of the skin in particular [2] Corticosteroids may predispose to dermatoporosis or aggravate preexisting dermatoporosis [1,2]. Dissecting hematomas of the skin may be precipitated by anticoagulant or corticosteroid therapy, as our patient was receiving. Corticosteroids are known to regulate the expression of genes encoding collagens I, III, IV, V, decorin, elastin, matrix metalloproteinases 1, 2, 3, tenascin as well as tissue inhibitors of certain matrix metalloproteinases [3]. In the presence of dermatoporosis, minimal trauma can cause massive bleeding into the virtual space between the dermis and subcutaneous adipose tissue or the subcutaneous adipose layer and the muscle fascia. The evolving hematoma destroys the blood supply to the skin and causes necrosis. In such situation immediate surgical evacuation of the hematoma and necrotic tissues should be performed to avoid extensive skin damage. Large and deep excisions may be necessary. The re-epithelization of larger defective skin surfaces may then be achieved by vacuum-assisted closure or autologous thin skin grafts. Dissecting hematomas result in long and costly hospital stays.

The final diagnosis in our patient was dermatoporosis and dissecting hematoma of the skin, predisposed by anticoagulant and corticosteroid treatment was. Three months later the ulcer as well as the minute skin lesions were healed.

Learning points:

- Atypical skin ulcers may pose challenging diagnostic problems.
- A spectrum of vasculopathies, infections affecting the skin, ulcerated neoplasms, panniculitis and neutrophilic dermatoses should be considered in the differential diagnosis.

- Atypical ischemic ulcerations of the extremity are often non-atherosclerotic in etiology, may involve the proximal segments, and can evolve despite palpable distal pulses.
- A high index of suspicion is required to recognize atypical pyoderma gangrenosum in an older adult.
- Among the clinical manifestations of skin aging, dissecting skin hematomas cause significant morbidity needing hospitalization and urgent surgical procedures.

Chronic leg ulceration is a common condition often present in patient admitted to the geriatric ward. Four etiologies are responsible for the large majority of skin ulcers in the elderly: trauma, ischemia, venous stasis and neuropathy. In a minority of cases, skin ulcers are manifestations of other diverse disease states. The above presented case history illustrates how important it is that physicians are aware of the different patterns of skin ulcers. Acute admissions are opportunities for detailed examination of ulcers in their clinical context, to consider further investigations and specialized treatment if needed.

References

[1] Saurat, H. Dermatoporosis. The functional side of skin aging. *Dermatology.,* 2007, 215, 271-272.

[2] Kaya, G, Saurat, JH. Dermatoporosis: A chronic cutaneous insufficiency/fragility syndrome. Clinicopathological features, mechanisms, prevention and potential treatments. *Dermatology.,* 2007, 215, 284-294.

[3] Schoepe, S; Schacke, H; May, E; Asadullah, K. Glucocorticoid therapy-induced skin atrophy. *Exp. Dermatol.,* 2006, 15, 406-420.

[4] Tomic-Canic, M; Brem, H. Gene array technology and pathogenesis of chronic wounds. *Am. J. Surg.,* 2004, 188 (1A suppl), 67-72.

[5] Robert, L; Labat-Robert, J. Aging of connective tissues: from genetic to epigenetic mechanisms. *Biogerontology*., 2000, 1, 123-131.

[6] Bello, YM; Phillips, TJ. Chronic leg ulcers: types and treatment. *Hosp. Pract.* (Minneap). 2000, Feb 15, 35(2), 101-107.

[7] Jaul, E. Non-healing wounds: The geriatric approach. *Arch. Gerontol. Geriatr.,* 2008 Oct 4. [Epub ahead of print].

[8] Levi, B; Rees, R. Diagnosis and management of pressure ulcers. *Clin. Plast. Surg.* 2007, 34, 735-748.

[9] Pataky, Z; Vischer, U. Diabetic foot disease in the elderly. *Diabetes Metab.,* 2007, Apr, 33 Suppl 1, S56-65.

[10] Tam, M; Moschella, SL.Vascular skin ulcers of limbs. *Cardiol. Clin.,* 1991, 9, 555-563.

[11] Nelzén, O; Bergqvist, D; Lindhagen, A. Venous and non-venous leg ulcers: clinical history and appearance in a population study. *Br. J. Surg.,* 1994, 81, 182-187.

[12] Singh, N; Armstrong, DG; Lipsky, BA. *JAMA.,* 2005, 293, 217-228.

[13] Garcia, AD; David, DR. Assessment and Management of Chronic Pressure Ulcers in the Elderly. *Medical Clinics of North America*., 2006, 90 (September):

[14] Grey, JE; Harding, KG; Enoch, S. Pressure ulcers. *BMJ.,* 2006, 332, 472-475.

[15] Reddy, M; Gill, SS; Rochon, PA. Preventing Pressure Ulcers: A Systematic Review. *JAMA.,* 2006, 296, 974-984.

[16] Palfreyman, SJ; Nelson, EA; Lochiel, R; Michaels, JA. Dressings for healing venous leg ulcers. *Cochrane Database Syst. Rev.,* 2006, 3, CD001103.

[17] Palfreyman, S, Nelson, EA, Michaels, JA. Dressings for venous leg ulcers: systematic review and meta-analysis. *BMJ.,* 2007, 335, 244.

[18] Howard, DP; Howard, A; Kothari, A; Wales, L; Guest, M; Davies, AH. The role of superficial venous surgery in the management of venous ulcers: a systematic review. *Eur. J. Vasc. Endovasc. Surg.,* 2008, 36, 458-465.

[19] Robson, MC; Cooper, DM; Aslam, R; Gould, LJ; Harding, KG; Margolis, DJ; Ochs, DE; Serena, TE; Snyder, RJ; Steed, DL; Thomas, DR; Wiersma-Bryant, L. Guidelines for the treatment of venous ulcers. *Wound Repair Regen.,* 2006, 14, 649-662.

[20] Lorentzen, HF. Clinical assessment of infection in nonhealing ulcers analyzed by latent class analysis. *Wound Repair Regen.,* 2006, 14, 350-353

[21] Slater, RA; Lazarovitch, T; Boldur, I; Ramot, Y; Buchs, A; Weiss, M; Hindi, A; Rapoport, MJ. Swab cultures accurately identify bacterial pathogens in diabetic foot wounds not involving bone. *Diabet. Med.* 2004, 21, 705-709.

[22] Schmidt, K; Debus, ES; St Jessberger Ziegler, U; Thiede, A. Bacterial population of chronic crural ulcers: is there a difference between the diabetic, the venous, and the arterial ulcer? *Vasa.*, 2000, 29, 62-70.

[23] Davies, CE. A prospective study of the microbiology of chronic venous leg ulcers to reevaluate the clinical predictive value of tissue biopsies and swabs. *Wound Repair Regen.*, 2007, 15, 17-22

[24] O'Meara, S. Antibiotics and antiseptics for venous leg ulcers. - *Cochrane Database Syst. Rev.*, 01-JAN-2008 (1).

[25] Butalia, S; Palda, VA; Sargeant, RJ; Detsky, AS; Mourad, O. Does This Patient With Diabetes Have Osteomyelitis of the Lower Extremity? *JAMA.*, 2008, 299, 806-813.

[26] Ford, CN; Reinhard, ER; Yeh, D; Syrek, D; De Las Morenas, A; Bergman, SB; Williams, S; Hamori, CA. Interim analysis of a prospective, randomized trial of vacuum-assisted clsoure versus the healthpoint system in the management of pressure ulcers. *Ann. Plast. Surg.*, 2002, 49, 55-61.

[27] Lipsky, BA; Berendt, AR; Deery, HG; Embil, JM; Joseph, WS; Karchmer, AW; et al., Infectious Disease Society of America (IDSA) Guidelines: Diagnosis and treatment of diabetic foot infections. *Clin. Infect. Dis.*, 2004, 39, 885-910.

[28] International Working Group on the Diabetic Foot (IWDGF). International Consensus on the Diabetic Foot (CD-ROM). Brussels: International Working Group on the Diabetic Foot (IWDGF), 2003.

[29] Castonguay, G. Short-stretch or four-layer compression bandages: an overview of the literature. *Ostomy Wound Manage.*, 2008, 54, 50-55.

[30] Singer, AJ; Dagum, AB. Current management of acute cutaneous wounds. *N. Engl. J. Med.*, 2008 , 359, 1037-1046.

[31] Vaneau, M; Chaby, G; Guillot, B; Martel, P; Senet, P; Téot, L; Chosidow, O. Consensus panel recommendations for chronic and acute wound dressings. *Arch. Dermatol.*, 2007, 143, 1291-1294.

[32] Livesley, NJ; Chow, AW. Infected pressure ulcers in elderly individuals. *Clin. Infect. Dis.*, 2002, 35, 1390-1396.

[33] Herschthal, J; Kirsner, RS. Current management of venous ulcers: an evidence-based review. *Surg. Technol. Int.*, 2008, 17, 77-83.

[34] Hinchliffe, RJ; Valk, GD; Apelqvist, J; Armstrong, DG; Bakker, K; Game, FL; Hartemann-Heurtier, A; Löndahl, M; Price, PE; van Houtum, WH; Jeffcoate, WJ. A systematic review of the effectiveness of interventions to enhance the healing of chronic ulcers of the foot in diabetes. *Diabetes Metab. Res. Rev.*, 2008, 24 Suppl 1, S119-44.

[35] Thackham, JA; McElwain, DL; Long, RJ. The use of hyperbaric oxygen therapy to treat chronic wounds: A review. *Wound Repair Regen.*, 2008, 16, 321-330.

[36] Ubbink, DT; Westerbos, SJ; Nelson, EA; Vermeulen, H. A systematic review of topical negative pressure therapy for acute and chronic wounds. *Br. J. Surg.,* 2008, 95, 685-692.

[37] Gregor, S; Maegele, M; Sauerland, S; Krahn, JF; Peinemann, F; Lange S. Negative pressure wound therapy: a vacuum of evidence? *Arch. Surg.,* 2008, 143, 189-196.

[38] Bazari, H; Jaff, MR; Mannstadt, M; Yan, S. Case records of the Massachusetts General Hospital. Case 7-2007. A 59-year-old woman with diabetic renal disease and nonhealing skin ulcers. *N. Engl. J. Med.,* 2007, 356, 1049-1057.

[39] Khorvash, F; Naeini, AE; Behjati, M; Karimifar, M; Khorvash, F; Dialami, K. Rapidly evolving purpuric lesions to massive hemorrhagic bullae, with rapid improvement by prednisolone: as a cutaneous manifestation of systemic lupus erythematosus: a case report. *Cases J.,* 2008, 1, 79.

[40] Naschitz, JE; Fields, M; Isseroff, H; Wolffson, V; Yeshurun, D. Unilateral necrobiosis lipoidica of the ischemic limb - a case report. *Angiology.,* 2003, 54, 239-242.

[41] Schneider, JW; Jordaan, HF. The histopathologic spectrum of erythema induratum of Bazin. *Am. J. Dermatopathol.,* 1997, 19, 323-333.

[42] Frantzeskaki, F; Betrosian, AP. Ecthyma gangrenosum: a rare manifestation of Pseudomonas aeruginosa sepsis in a critically ill adult patient. *Eur. J. Dermatol.,* 2008, 18, 345-346.

[43] Weir, E. Buruli ulcer: the third most common mycobacterial infection. *CCMAJ.,* 2002, 166, 1691.

[44] Daudén, E; Oñate, MJ. Calciphylaxis. *Dermatol. Clin.,* 2008, 26, 557-568.

[45] Weidmann, A; Harkins, K. What lies beneath? Assessment of leg ulcers during acute hospital admission. *Age Ageing.*, 2008, 37, 117-118.

[46] Meenakshisundaram, S; Myint, PK. Atypical pyoderma gangrenosum in an older adult: high index of suspicion is required. *Age Ageing.,* 20051, 34, 422.

[47] Dean, SM. Atypical ischemic lower extremity ulcerations: a differential diagnosis. *Vasc. Med.,* 2008, 13, 47-54.

[48] Bennett, ML; Jackson, JM; Jorizzo, JL; Fleischer, AB; Jr, White, WL; Callen, JP. Pyoderma gangrenosum. A comparison of typical and

atypical forms with an emphasis on time to remission. Case review of 86 patients from 2 institutions. *Medicine.* (Baltimore), 2000, 79, 37-46.

[49] Callen, JP; Jackson, JM. Pyoderma gangrenosum: an update. *Rheum. Dis. Clin. North Am.,* 2007,33, 787-802.

[50] De la Morena, F; Martín, L; Gisbert, JP; Fernández Herrera, J; Goiriz, R. Refractory and infected pyoderma gangrenosum in a patient with ulcerative colitis: response to infliximab. *Inflamm. Bowel Dis.,* 2007, 13, 509-510.

[51] Wollina, U. Clinical management of pyoderma gangrenosum. *Am. J. Clin. Dermatol.,* 2002, 3, 149-158.

In: Ulcers: Causes, Diagnosis, and Treatment ISBN: 978-1-60741-253-3
Editors: Danijel Erceg et al. pp. 89-100

Chapter 7

TOPICALLY APPLIED MORPHINE GEL FOR PAINFUL ULCERS

Quy N.H. Tran*
Department of Internal Medicine
University of California at Davis, Medical Center
Sacramento, CA 95817, USA

ABSTRACT

Although it has been well established that opioid analgesics relieve pain by acting on receptors in the central nervous system, research has suggested that similar analgesia can be achieved through peripheral opioid receptors. Basic science research has demonstrated that malignant or benign skin ulcers can expose peripheral sensory nerve terminals, while local inflammation within the ulcer up-regulates opioid receptors. Thus, one strategy to manage pain arising from these ulcers would be to apply topical opioid agonists, usually in the form of a gel. While systemic absorption likely varies with extent of ulceration, topical analgesics could reduce the need for systemic medications and the resultant adverse effects. However, research in the area has been slow; a few small randomized trials and case series suggest benefits from morphine gel. Whether it is a placebo effect or actual analgesia produced from

* Corresponding Author: Dr. Quy Tran, University of California at Davis, Medical Center, 4150 V Street, PSSB Suite 3100, Sacramento, CA 95817, E-mail: quy.tran@ucdmc.ucdavis.edu.

peripheral receptors, many unfortunate patients suffer from difficult to treat ulcerative pain and may appear to benefit from a topical strategy. Larger studies are needed and, fortunately, are being conducted to help establish topical opioid therapy as a viable adjunct to systemic therapy in treating pain from ulcers.

INTRODUCTION

Opioid analgesics relieve pain by acting on receptors in the central nervous system, often at the expense of significant side effects. Research has suggested that similar analgesia can be achieved through peripheral receptors through a neuroimmune pathway. Light microscopic techniques have demonstrated opioid receptors in the periphery of fine cutaneous nerves and, depending on particular circumstances, sensory axons can be immunostained for mu-, delta-, or kappa-receptors [1, 2]. These opioid receptors are quiescent and are difficult to find in normal tissue, but are detectable after peripheral injury and onset of inflammation. With pronounced inflammation, the perineurium is disrupted, exposing the receptors to potential opioid agonists, while also creating an environment to enhance their efficacy. These activated receptors may be stimulated by mechanical, chemical, or thermal means. In addition, inflammation promotes distal transport of these receptors along the axon to the periphery further concentrating the number of available and active receptors [3]. Immune cells within inflamed subcutaneous tissue can synthesize and release endogenous opioid peptides that interact with these receptors. This interaction alters potassium and calcium currents within the neurons that can cause inhibition of neuronal excitation, action potential propagation, and release of proinflammatory peptides, thereby producing analgesia [4]. Interestingly, similar effects can be produced with exogenous opioid agonists and the analgesia can be reversed with naloxone.

Because of these findings, there has been interest in using opioid agonists in patients with benign or malignant ulcers. Pain arising from these ulcers is often difficult to treat and it is common for patients to continue to experience pain despite using systemic medications. The destructive nature of these ulcers exposes cutaneous nerves that could potentially be a target for locally applied opioid agonists. The strategy of using locally-acting analgesia has the advantage of low systemic bioavailability and potentially decreased related adverse effects. Patients could conceivably achieve greater analgesia while taking fewer or lower doses of oral medications and thus reduce the risk of sedation, respiratory depression, nausea and constipation. Several clinical trials and case series have reported good analgesia with few side effects using topical morphine in the treatment of painful ulcers. In this chapter, two patients with painful ulcers (one with malignant ulcers, the other with benign ulcers) treated with topical morphine gel are discussed followed by a review of the available literature regarding this modality of treatment.

First Case

A 52-year-old man with Stage IIb mycosis fungoides was admitted for pain control. His pain arose from skin lesions that were in varying stages of healing. As an outpatient, he was initially started on hydrocodone as needed and was quickly titrated up to long-acting morphine with liquid short-acting morphine as needed. About one month before his admission, his long-acting morphine was converted to methadone 30 mg orally three times a day. On the day of admission, he reported that he self-titrated his methadone dose to 50 mg orally three times a day and continued to use short-acting morphine for breakthrough pain. This regimen did not provide significant relief. He also noted that the pain medications affected his concentration, were quite sedating, and caused severe dose-limiting constipation. In addition, prior treatment with diverse chemotherapy regimens offered minimal resolution of his primary disease, and so, he continued to experience considerable pain. Given the chronic and progressive nature of his disease, his physical exam was notable for widespread skin lesions, which ranged from mild erythematous patches to scaly plaques to open weeping ulcers, covering his entire body. To control his pain, he was continued on his previously prescribed dose of methadone at 30 mg orally three times a day and started on a patient controlled analgesia (PCA) pump to calculate his additional needs.

Despite increasing analgesic dosing with the PCA, he continued to experience pain. By the fifth day of his admission, his PCA was discontinued and he was started on oxycodone 5-20 mg orally every 6 hours as needed. His pain continued. On hospital day seven, the methadone was increased to 40 mg orally three times a day and oxycodone was increased to 5-30 mg orally every 4 hours as needed. Pain control remained inadequate. On the eighth day of his admission, with his consent, a trial of topical opioids was initiated. A mixture of 10 mg of morphine sulfate injection was combined with 8 grams of a neutral water-based gel. A test dose applied to a small patch of skin was well tolerated. The patient then applied the morphine gel to five or six of the larger (greater than 2.5 cm in diameter) and more painful lesions. Under the guidance of a wound care nurse, he liberally applied the morphine gel to each lesion 2-3 times per day as needed. Before the utilization of morphine gel, the patient's pain scores ranged from 5-10 (on a scale from 0-10 with 10 being the worse pain) with most scores around 7. With the addition of morphine gel, his pain scores ranged from 0-9 with almost half of his scores under 5. He was discharged with satisfactory pain relief two days later on a regimen of morphine gel applied 2-3 times daily as needed, methadone 40 mg orally three times a day for basal pain control and oxycodone 5-30 mg orally every 4 hours as needed for breakthrough pain. He was admitted several more times over the next several months and continued to require higher doses of narcotics. He died 5 months later due to his progressive, uncontrolled disease.

Second Case

A 55-year-old sedentary woman with diabetes mellitus type 2 and stage III-IV bilateral lower extremity and decubitus ulcers was admitted to the surgical team for debridement of these ulcers. The medicine service was consulted to assist in managing the patient's diabetes and to recommend a medication regimen to help control the pain arising from these ulcers. As an outpatient, she was started on hydrocodone as needed for pain. As her ulcerative disease progressed, the pain worsened, and she was titrated to a regimen of extended release oxycodone 20 mg orally two times a day with hydrocodone as needed for pain. When she was admitted, she was continued on her extended release oxycodone and given morphine sulfate injections every two hours as needed for pain. Her pain scores ranged from 5-10 (on a scale from 0-10 with 10 being the worse pain), with higher numbers corresponding to dressing changes.

Because of the localizing nature of her pain, it was felt that a topical strategy for pain control would benefit her. With her consent, a trial of morphine gel was initiated. A mixture of 10 mg of morphine sulfate injection was combined with 10 grams of a neutral water-based gel. A test dose applied to a small patch of skin was well tolerated, so the patient self-applied the morphine gel to all of her lesions. Under the guidance of a wound care nurse, she liberally applied the morphine gel to each lesion 2-3 times per day as needed. She continued to have pain with scores ranging from 3-6, but she noted that this range was tolerable for her. She was titrated off the extended release oxycodone and only used morphine gel and as needed hydrocodone during the hospital course. She was discharged in good condition on this regimen.

CONCLUSION

The management of pain due to malignant or benign skin ulcers is of great importance. The number of patients who suffer from benign ulcers, including those with pressure ulcers or ulcers that develop as a result of long-standing diabetes mellitus or peripheral vascular disease is tremendous. Approximately 26% of hospice patients[5] and as many as 40,000 patients per year suffer from pain due to pressure ulcers and thousands more suffer from ulcers due to chronic medical conditions.[6] In addition, ulcers that develop from malignant etiologies such as Kaposi's sarcoma, melanoma, breast cancer, rectal cancer or mycosis fungoides, cause pain and suffering to an unfortunate patient population. The issue of adequate analgesia in these patients is difficult and the strategy of using topically applied agents may provide another form of pain relief.

Most studies on topically applied opioids to treat pain that arise from ulcers use a mixture of 10 mg of morphine sulfate combined with 8 g of a neutral water based gel (typically Intrasite® gel, Smith and Nephew Healthcare Ltd, Middlesex, UK), although other doses of morphine, alternative narcotics (such as methadone powder[7]) and other gels and delivery systems (such as metronidazole gel[8], silver sulphadiazine cream[9], and Stomahesive® powder[7]), have been utilized. Systemic absorption of morphine gel likely varies with extent of ulceration. When applied to cutaneous ulcers, one study noted that morphine and its metabolites, morphine-6-glucuronide (M6G) and morphine-3-glucuronide (M3G), were undetectable in the plasma of most patients.[10] The same study also noted that in one patient with a large surface area ulcer, morphine, M6G, and M3G were all detected in the plasma. In this patient, morphine and M6G bioavailability were 20% and 21%, respectively, while M3G was below the lower limit of quantification. Thus, systemic absorption for the majority of patients is negligible, which would lead to the decreased likelihood of systemic adverse effects.

Several years after basic science research demonstrated analgesic actions of exogenous opioids in peripheral tissue, case series began to appear in the literature. Jepson reported a series of 17 patients with 30 ulcers and used topical benzydamine in an aqueous solution.[11] Within the first 24 hours, significant pain relief was reported in 29 of 30 ulcers. Pain relief was achieved in all ulcers by 48 hours. Back *et al.* reported using diamorphine in Intrasite gel in three patients with skin ulcers and was able to produce adequate analgesia in these patients within 72 hours.[12] In a descriptive case series, Twillman *et al.* reported on nine consecutive patients treated with morphine-infused gel dressing.[6] Eight patients had open ulcers: three patients with decubitus ulcers, three patients with ulcers arising from chronic medical conditions, and two patients with malignant ulcers. The ninth patient had colorectal cancer and pain due to swelling and inflammation of his scrotum, but had no open wounds. All patients were treated with either a 0.1% or a 0.15% weight-to-weight concentration of morphine gel and seven of nine patients experienced substantial pain relief, one patient experienced some pain relief, and the patient without an open wound did not experience any relief.

Based on these promising observational studies, two small randomized, double-blind, placebo-controlled, crossover pilot studies were conducted.[13, 14] Published simultaneously, the first study recruited 13 patients in a palliative care setting with painful grade II or III pressure ulcers to be treated with a 0.1% weight-to-weight mixture of a diamorphine gel.[13] The six patients that did not complete the study died either before or during the trial or developed confusion necessitating withdrawal from the trial. The patients were randomly assigned to either three days of placebo gel followed by diamorphine gel or vice versa. Pain scores improved significantly 1 and 12 hours after application of diamorphine gel as compared to placebo gel. In the other study, five patients with painful sacral ulcers were first treated with either morphine gel or placebo for two days.[14] After a two-day washout, patients were crossed over for a further two days of the alternative treatment. Patients completed a visual analogue scale (VAS) twice daily, with lower numbers indicating more pain relief. Mean VAS scores for patients during placebo was 47 ± 11 and during morphine was 15 ± 11. There was no difference in the use of rescue medications during either treatment arm. Adverse effects included itching, burning or discomfort, but these effects occurred in both arms and none could be directly attributed to the morphine. Intrasite gel is generally well tolerated, but it is also used for debridement of necrotic tissue, thus some of the adverse effects noted could be attributed to the natural action of the hydrogel. A larger, follow-up randomized, double-blind, placebo-controlled study included 16 patients, 13 with pressure ulcers and 3 with malignant ulcers.[15] Analgesia was rated using a numerical rating score (NRS) with lower numbers indicating more pain relief. Mean NRS scores during pretreatment, with morphine, and with placebo were 6.6 ± 1.6, 2.8 ± 1.3, and 5.5 ± 1.9, respectively. Similar adverse effects were noted in the larger study. Because of these results, Porzio *et al.* encouraged further research and reported their own case series of three patients with pressure sores and two patients with malignant ulcers treated with morphine gel and reported significant pain relief in all five patients.[16] Similarly, Abbas reported a series of 17 patients with grade 2+ pressure ulcers treated with diamorphine gel and mean VAS scores improved from 9.4 to 4.6 after treatment.[17]

Topical morphine gel is not limited to use in the adult population and small case series are beginning to appear in the pediatric literature. Use of morphine gel in the pediatric population with painful inflammatory skin lesions would prove advantageous since the use of systemic opioids are often limited by frequent side effects experienced by young patients. In one study, two pediatric patients with epidermolysis bullosa with painful denuded areas of skin resulting from recurring bullae formation were treated with morphine gel.[18] The morphine gel mixture consisted of 10 mg of morphine sulfate with 15 g of Intrasite gel with the dose of morphine at 0.2 mg/kg. One patient had a 40-55% reduction in pain scores; the other patient who was opioid naïve had a 66% reduction in the pain score. To date, both patients have not reported any adverse side effects.

Expanding on the data collected for the treatment of cutaneous ulcers using topically applied opioids, several researchers have utilized locally applied exogenous opioids to treat the pain associated with esophageal and mucosal damage due to chemoradiotherapy. Gairard-Dory *et al.* used a slightly modified morphine gel for patients suffering from esophagitis.[19] They reported on three patients with non-small cell lung cancer treated with 36 Gy of radiotherapy and all patients subsequently experienced at least grade III radiotherapy-induced esophagitis. Instead of using Intrasite gel, morphine sulfate was mixed with a ready-mixed Purilon gel, and the patients swallowed 2 to 10 mL of 0.1% of this morphine gel. All patients reported pain relief with the morphine gel. One patient reported nausea with the mixture, which was corrected by having the patient take small amounts. No other adverse effects were reported. Cerchietti *et al.* did not utilize a morphine gel mixture in their study of mucositis-associated pain from chemoradiotherapy, but used a morphine mouthwash and compared it to a magic mouthwash comprised of aluminum hydroxide, viscous lidocaine and diphenhydramine. All twenty six patients had either grade 2 or 3 mucositis. The 14 patients assigned to the morphine mouthwash arm reported a significant decrease in pain scores, a longer duration of pain relief and a shorter duration of severe functional impairment.[20] Only one patient in this arm experienced local side effects. Esophagitis and mucositis are often the dose limiting toxicity associated with chemoradiotherapy with few options to utilize in treating pain associated with these inflammatory conditions. Based on these studies, topical opioids provide an attractive alternative or adjunct to traditional therapy.

In Practice

These case series and randomized controlled trials have all suggested that morphine gel is beneficial and efficacious, but the studies are small and no large definitive trials have been conducted. It is likely that morphine gel will not supplant the use of oral analgesics in the treatment of pain arising from ulcers, but experience has shown that it can be used as a successful adjunct to such therapy. In these two sample patients, morphine gel provided additional pain relief and worked in conjunction with the primary strategy of oral analgesics. Both patients reported that the morphine gel allowed them to rest at night and made dressing changes more tolerable, but both relied on oral medications as their main form of analgesia. Given the lessons learned from these and other similar patients, some institutions have begun to use morphine gel in patients with ulcer pain that is not controlled with oral analgesics alone.

Despite the lack of large trials, these smaller studies do yield promising results for the large patient population that suffers from pain arising from ulcers. Morphine gel may provide an effective and relatively safe modality to relieve pain. Morphine gel can readily be prepared by any compounding pharmacy. The choice of hydrogel to use is dependent on the pharmacy's formulary, but should be one in which the hydrogel is chemically stable and inert. The morphine component of the compound has been shown to be stable for up to 28 days when mixed with a neutral water based hydrogel with no detectable break down products.[21] If mixed under sterile conditions, it can be used safely for 28 days. If morphine gel is mixed under non-sterile conditions, due to infection control concerns, the mixture should be used within seven days. A month's supply can conveniently be prescribed and safely used if stored below 25°C in a dry place. Few adverse effects have been reported, but care needs to be exercised in patients with sensitivities to any component of morphine gel. Common adverse events reported in our patients are similar to reported case series and include itching and skin irritation, likely due to debriding action of the hydrogel. Systemic side effects are very rare, so patient adherence is high. Some patients have noted that morphine gel can be messy, but this can be minimized with gauze wraps. Abuse potential is low because of the difficulty in separating the morphine sulfate from the gel once it is mixed, but vigilance is recommended in prescribing large quantities of morphine gel.

Basic and clinical research supports the use of morphine gel, but the widespread utilization in actual clinical practice has been slow. Based on these promising studies, any patient presenting with pain of primarily ulcer origin should be evaluated for morphine gel therapy. Many treatment algorithms exist for treating patients with painful ulcers and morphine gel should be a component of these algorithms. Usually, patients can be started on morphine gel as an adjunctive therapy when patients continue to have pain despite increasing doses of oral medications or experience significant side effects from those medications. A starting concentration of 10 mg of morphine sulfate with 10 gm of a hydrogel can be initially tried and although there is no known maximum dose, most studies report achieving an effect before reaching a concentration of 10 mg of morphine sulfate with 5 gm of a hydrogel dosed at three times a day. No studies have looked at the amount of gel to apply to each wound and the dwell time the mixture should stay on the wounds. Most patients apply either a thin film or the minimum amount of morphine gel necessary to just cover the wound, and leave the mixture on until the next dressing change. Nursing protocols to utilize morphine gel can be adapted from standard wound care protocols. Caution is advised with stage IV ulcers as a minimum amount of morphine or its metabolites may be absorbed systemically. A slow titration schedule is recommended for these large and deep ulcers. Morphine gel applied to exudative wounds may be diluted or flushed away due to the extremely moist environment and dosing amounts and schedules should be adjusted to account for this.

FUTURE DIRECTIONS

Many patients would likely benefit from morphine gel, and larger clinical trials are beginning to appear to definitively establish efficacy. Trials utilizing morphine gel to treat pain arising from benign ulcers are currently underway, and trials focusing on malignant ulcers are being designed. Results of these larger trials should start to appear within the next couple of years. Trials examining whether morphine or its metabolites affect wound healing have not been conducted, and would be important to patients with benign ulcers, such as pressure ulcers, where wound healing is paramount. Duration of pain relief from morphine gel has not been well-studied and trials examining this would help in establishing proper dosing protocols. Currently, protocols are based on anecdotal evidence.

The fact that peripheral opioid receptors are active in inflamed tissue makes topical opioid therapy an attractive option in treating pain caused by many acute and subacute clinical scenarios, such as in post-operative wounds, vaginal or rectal fistulae, traumatic injuries, and arthritis. Combining an opioid with an antibiotic gel and affixing the mixture to a mesh would provide an appealing adjunctive solution to treating ulcers, wounds and injuries that are often painful and infected. This multimodality treatment strategy would allow convenient and rapid placement of local therapy at the site of the lesion. Fortunately, these trials and product developments are progressing quickly, making gel therapy a more attractive and viable option for patients and clinicians.

ACKNOWLEDGMENTS

This chapter was inspired by an article originally printed in The Journal of Supportive Oncology, parts of which are re-printed here with permission from Elsevier Science.

REFERENCES

[1] Coggeshall, RE; Zhou, S; Carlton, SM. Opioid receptors on peripheral sensory axons. *Brain Research,* 1997, 764(1-2), 126-32.

[2] Truong, W; Cheng, C; Xu, QG; Li, XQ; Zochodne, DW. Mu opioid receptors and analgesia at the site of a peripheral nerve injury. *Ann. Neurology,* 2003, 53(3), 366-75.

[3] Hassan, A; Ableitner, A; Stein, C; Herz, A. Inflammation of the rat paw enhanced axonal transport of opioid receptors in the sciatic nerve and increases their density in the inflamed tissue. *Neuroscience,* 1993, 55(1), 185-95.

[4] Stein, C. The control of pain in peripheral tissue by opioids. *NEJM,* 1995, 332(25), 1685-90.

[5] Galvin, J. An audit of pressure ulcer incidence in a palliative care setting. *Int. J. Palliat. Nurs.,* 2002, 8(5), 214-21.

[6] Twillman, R; Long, TD; Cathers, TA; Mueller, DW. Treatment of painful skin ulcers with topical opioids. *J. Pain Symptom Manage,* 1999, 17(4), 288-92.

[7] Gallagher, RE; Arndt, DR; Hunt, KL. Analgesic effects of topical methadone - a report of four cases. *Clin. J. Pain,* 2005, 21(2), 190-2.

[8] Flock, P; Gibbs, L; Sykes, N. Diamorphine-metronidazole gel effective for treatment of painful infected leg ulcers. *J. Pain Symptom Manage,* 2000, 20(6), 396-7.

[9] Krajnik, M; Zylicz, Z; Finlay, I; Luczak, J; Sorge, AAv. Potential uses of topical opioids in palliative care - report of 6 cases. *Pain,* 1999, 80(1999).

[10] Ribeiro, MDC; Joel, SP; Zeppetella, G. The bioavailability of morphine applied topically to cutaneous ulcers. *J. Pain Symptom Manage,* 2004, 27(5), 434-9.

[11] Jepson, BA. Relieving the pain of pressure sores. The Lancet 1992, 339(8791), 503-4.

[12] Back, IN; Findlay, I. Analgesic effect of topical opioids on painful skin ulcers. *J. Pain Symptom Manage,* 1995, 10(7), 493.

[13] Flock, P. Pilot study to determine the effectiveness of diamorphine gel to control pressure ulcer pain. *J. Pain Symptom Manage, 2*003, 25(6), 547-54.

[14] Zeppetella, G; Paul, J; Ribeiro, MDC. Analgesic efficacy of morphine applied topically to painful ulcers. *J. Pain Symptom Manage,* 2003, 25(6), 555-8.

[15] Zeppetella, G; Ribeiro, MDC. Morphine in Intrasite gel applied topically to painful ulcers. *J. Pain Symptom Manage,* 2005, 29(2), 118-9.

[16] Porzio, G; Aielli, F; Verna, L; Cannita, K; Marchetti, P; Ficorella, C. Topical morphine in the treatment of painful ulcers. *J. Pain Symptom Manage,* 2005, 30(4), 304-5.

[17] Abbas, SQ. Diamorphine-Intrasite dressings for painful pressure ulcers. *J. Pain Symptom Manage,* 2004, 28(6), 532-4.

[18] Watterson, G; Howard, R; Goldman, A. Peripheral opioids in inflammatory pain. *Arch. Dis. Child,* 2004, 89(7), 679-81.

[19] Gairard-Dory, AC; Schaller, C; Mennecier, B; et al. Chemoradiotherapy-induced esophagitis pain relieved by topical morphine: three cases. *J. Pain Symptom Manage,* 2005, 30(2), 107-9.

[20] Cerchietti, LCH; Navigante, AH; Bonomi, MR; et al. Effect of topical morphine for mucositis-associated pain following concomitant

chemoradiotherapy for head and neck carcinoma. *Cancer* 2002, 95(10), 2230-6.

[21] Zeppetella, G; Joel, SP; Ribeiro, MDC. Stability of morphine sulphate and diamorphine hydrochloride in Intrasite gel. *Palliative Medicine,* 2005, 19, 131-6.

CHAPTER SOURCES

Chapter 4 was also published in Smoking and Womens Health, edited by Merideth K. Wesley and Ingrid A. Sternbach, Nova Science Publishers. It was submitted for appropriate modifications in an effort to encourage wider dissemination of research.

Chapter 6 was also published in Challenges in Acute Geriatric Care, edited/authored by Jochannan E. Naschitz, Nova Science Publishers. It was submitted for appropriate modifications in an effort to encourage wider dissemination of research.

Chapter 7 was also published in Pain Management: New Research, edited by Paolo S. Grecoard and Francesco M. Conti, Nova Science Publishers. It was submitted for appropriate modifications in an effort to encourage wider dissemination of research.

IDNEX

A

B

C

E

F

G

H

I

J

K

L

M

N

O

P

N

O

P

Q

R

S

T

U

V

W

X

Y